It's an... ...n
the da... ...st
produc... ...t,
then y...

Now is the time to take back your life with

SAY GOODBYE TO BACK PAIN

From symptoms to diagnosis to cure, you'll find trustworthy,
up-to-date information on many common causes of pain,
including

muscle spasm · herniated disk

torn disks · whiplash

spinal narrowing · spinal slippage

osteoporosis · osteoarthritis

benign and malignant tumors · sciatica

inflammatory diseases · infection

And you'll discover treatment options you may not have
known were available to you, from nonmedical approaches
to the very latest in surgical technology.

Why "live" with back pain—when you can control or
even prevent the problems you may have thought you had to
endure for life?

W9-BEX-340

Also by Marian Betancourt

*What's in the Air? The Complete Guide to
Seasonal and Year-Round Airborne Allergies*
(with Gillian Shepherd, M.D.)

Published by Pocket Books

Say Goodbye to Back Pain

Emile Hiesiger, M.D., and Marian Betancourt

POCKET BOOKS
New York London Toronto Sydney

An *Original* Publication of POCKET BOOKS

POCKET BOOKS, a division of Simon & Schuster, Inc.
1230 Avenue of the Americas, New York, NY 10020

ISBN: 978-1-4767-9277-4

First Pocket Books printing October 2004

10 9 8 7 6 5 4 3 2 1

POCKET and colophon are registered trademarks of Simon & Schuster, Inc.

Front cover photo © Taxi/Eric O'Connell

Manufactured in the United States of America

For information regarding special discounts for bulk purchases, please contact Simon & Schuster Special Sales at 1-800-456-6798 or business@simonandschuster.com

This book is for my father for his support and understanding over the years. I also dedicate it to my patients who have taught me more about pain than any textbook, lecture, or professor, and to Howard C. Baron, M.D., who introduced me to the profession and the challenges of vascular surgery. The sections on spinal surgery and tumors are dedicated to a senior colleague and dear friend, Dr. Vallo Benjamin, a truly brilliant neurosurgeon who has patiently and constructively taught me more about the diagnosis and treatment of spinal disorders than anyone else.

E.H.

As always, this is dedicated to my family, a constant source of love and support.

M.B.

ACKNOWLEDGMENTS

I am fortunate to be surrounded by people who are interested in this book and who helped make it possible. In addition to my friend and colleague, Dr. Vallo Benjamin, I owe thanks to William Breger, a longtime friend and outstanding architect, for critically reviewing the entire manuscript. Dr. Hal Mitnick, a senior professor of rheumatology at New York University Hospital and an invaluable colleague, made important suggestions regarding the sections on osteoporosis and benign medical diseases affecting the spine. Dr. Henry Birnbaum, a young colleague and skilled physiatrist, helped enormously with the physical therapy chapter, especially the section on spinal exercises. His encouragement and helpful criticisms of the entire manuscript were most appreciated. Also, thanks to my colleague Dr. Leslie St. Louis for allowing me to utilize his outstanding radiological facility for outpatient procedures. I am deeply indebted to him for critical assistance in preparing portions of this manuscript.

My office staff, headed by Judy Vargas, deserves extraordinary thanks. Without their remarkable patience, interest, and consideration, preparing this manuscript would have been far more torturous for me and distracting from the care of my patients. Ms. Vargas, out of tremendous loyalty and dedication, exhausted herself successfully running the business aspects of the office, while I at times neglected it, due to the exigencies of completing this book.

I especially thank my dear wife, Patricia, for her loving

viii   Acknowledgments

help and support and for putting up with the time constraints and anxiety imposed upon our relationship during the preparation of this book.

E.H.

Thanks to Christina Boys, an insightful and thoughtful editor, for her enthusiasm and professionalism. And to Nancy Love, a literary agent par excellence, for the same reasons.

M.B.

DISCLAIMER

This book is meant to educate readers about how the spine works and how to understand the causes of back pain and what can be done about it. It is designed to help readers get proper care and prevent further pain. It is not meant to replace medical treatment.

CONTENTS

INTRODUCTION

By the time people come to me with back pain, they have been to many other doctors and have been suffering for many years. Their pain has become the three-ton elephant in the room. Persistent back pain, the second most common human affliction after the common cold, affects 31 million Americans at any given time. Chronic, moderate-to-severe low back pain affects over two-thirds of patients enrolled in chronic-pain centers. Unfortunately, many Americans live in physical and often emotional agony from poorly controlled back pain. Because it can be hard to find the source of the pain, some doctors blame it on the patient's emotional problems. Unfortunately, the patients and their families believe this.

Diagnosis is an art as well as a science, and diagnosing back problems is challenging because the cause of the pain is often hidden and may not show up on X-rays or other scans. Pain travels along the complicated nervous system pathways, so the source of pain is often far from where it is perceived. Because chronic pain affects our emotions and everybody has a different pain threshold, this adds to the difficulty and frustration in finding treatment that works. When we cannot verify the presence of pain or measure its severity, the result is insufficient understanding and treatment by society, the medical profession, insurance companies, and the family and friends of the person in pain. *There is almost always a physical cause of back pain.* A conscientious doctor, willing to face the challenge with a cooperative patient, will almost always identify it.

Treatment for spinal pain should begin with the simplest, most conservative therapy before invasive therapy is even considered. For example, most herniated disks eventually shrink, and the pain and weakness or numbness they caused resolves. Yet far too many people are rushed into surgery. This often results in being married forever to the medical system and more spinal surgery. As you will see in this book, very few conditions warrant surgery.

The cause of back pain is often multifaceted and in many cases back pain can be relieved, lessened, or even prevented by changes in lifestyle. Weight loss, proper exercises, and posture, as well as good pain medication, should be used intelligently and creatively to maximize your pain relief before you consider any more invasive procedures. I know this is easier said than done, but it is not impossible. There is no reason for your aching spine to destroy you or your quality of life.

I am neither a proponent nor opponent of any medication, physical therapy, surgery, implantable devices, or anything else. There are many therapies to help you deal with chronic spinal pain, depending on the diagnosis and your personal situation. Diagnosis, not just pain management, is the key to successful treatment. Getting the correct diagnosis and subsequent high-quality treatment may well cost you money out of pocket, a very good reason not to allow yourself to go down the financial tube before getting yourself turned around with proper treatment. I want to liberate you from the pain clinic and medical system as much as possible so you can go on about whatever life you may have on this planet. We have all recently been reminded just how tenuous life can be. Live it to the fullest.

Throughout the book you will find stories of people who thought they would never get rid of their back pain—yet did. Because your spine is a living—and aging—part of your superstructure, it may cause pain again over the years. In my own case, as I sit for long hours at my desk writing this book under the stress of a deadline, *I have been doing everything I tell you* not *to do*. This stress and my minimally arthritic back have worked together to create back pain. However, despite minor arthritic changes in my spine, I don't always have back pain. My stress level fluctuates, as does strain on my back, while sitting for hours on end writing a manuscript or standing still slightly bent over a patient for long periods of time during a difficult procedure.

I hope this book will take some of the mystery out of why your back hurts and what you can do about it. By learning exactly how your spine, muscles, and nerves work, you will gain insight into how they can be damaged or cause pain.

The first part of the book is meant to enlighten you about your spinal anatomy, how to get your pain properly diagnosed, and how to find the right doctor and treatment.

The second part examines the most common sources of back pain and how they should—and should not—be treated.

And, finally, there is a chapter on prevention, so you can avoid future back pain at home or at work or away. There are key points at the end of each chapter to help you digest what you've learned.

E.H.

Part I

The Basics

The Mind-Body Connection
of Chronic Back Pain

The International Association for the Study of Pain defines pain as "an unpleasant sensory and emotional experience that we primarily associate with tissue damage or describe in terms of such damage." The definition of pain has two parts. One part deals with the sensation of tissue damage: A burn is perceived as different from a blow from a hammer to your thumb. Its intensity is rated, and it is localized. However, the experience of physical pain involves an emotional response to that injury, a feeling about its unpleasantness and a reaction to the pain. Those who have experienced extreme anxiety or depression recognize easily that mental dysfunction may also elicit an emotional response that is experienced as painful.

If you are under increasing levels of stress, you will be more sensitive to pain. If you twist a back muscle while picking up your child after an enjoyable weekend when you are well rested, it won't hurt much at all. But if you twist that same muscle with the same force after a stressful week at the office, when everything went wrong, you may find the pain excruciating. The same amount of "injury" is felt with a different intensity of pain. I learned this myself as I was writing this book in the final days against the deadline.

Pain signals the brain, and its perception as pain can be modified by a number of mechanisms. Our body produces its own narcotic-like pain relievers, endorphins. These chemicals block transmission of pain. Endorphins also are released by regular exercise. Feeling good and reducing stress also can release them.

When physical pain is long standing, it often results in psychological pain of anxiety and depression. People with chronic moderate-to-severe pain become irritable. Many become listless or depressed. Some feel useless and unable to cope. People have ruined their lives because they enter—or are forced into—a downward spiral of incorrect diagnoses, untreated pain, disability, depression, and more pain and suffering.

Most of my own patients are not disabled; I won't let them go out on permanent disability unless they have a condition that is likely to worsen with time, such as progressive cancer. This is not because I am cruel or dispassionate but because I am very aware of the economic, social, and psychological downfall of disability. Most Americans disabled for a year never return to work—or full enjoyment of life. And, as you know, life is not getting any easier or cheaper. Your disability payments of today may not be as helpful ten years from now. But in all likelihood you'll still be alive, in increasing financial distress, depressed, and in pain. Because of what chronic disability creates, you'll have less financial and logistical means of finding and using high-quality medical care, including new, improved, but invariably expensive drugs and other pain-relieving treatments.

I hope that this book will help you avoid or get off disability. Of the patients on temporary disability I have worked with, I have been able to put the overwhelming majority back to work, sometimes with a different job from the one they previously had. The vast majority don't even go on temporary disability.

Chapter 1

Understanding How
Your Back Works

You don't need to go through medical school, but a little knowledge about how your spine works may go a long way in helping you understand what can go wrong, what to do about it, when to see a specialist, and how to prevent pain. Your spine is your main means of support and keeps you upright. The ingenious design of this large organ includes bones, muscles, ligaments, and nerves. It's also the guardian of your spinal cord, which, along with your brain, makes up the central nervous system.

Your spine moves like a semirigid gooseneck lamp, with the greatest movement in your neck—which might move three hundred times a day—and your lower back, which supports the weight of the top half of your body as you bend and straighten up, rotate, and pick things up from the ground. The gooseneck shape serves an important purpose, curving to allow room for the heart and lungs in the chest while keeping the head centered over the lower body and the pelvis. This shape is well balanced, the structure strong.

Whether you run a marathon or pick a book up from the floor, the disks lying between the bones (vertebrae) of your spine absorb the shocks of pressure and cushion those bones to protect you from injury and pain. The wear and tear to the joints connecting these bones, the disks, and related structures is at the root of most back pain. Joints become arthritic, disks tear or protrude and press on a nerve, supporting ligaments harden, and so on. We can face these risks at any age. Young people as well as old can get muscle spasms, stress fractures, and a variety of sports injuries to the spine.

SPINAL BONES: VERTEBRAE

There are thirty-two horseshoe-shaped vertebrae in your spine. The vertebrae and interspersed disks not only support the weight of your spine; they protect your spinal cord. They are organized this way, starting at the top of the spine. (See figures 1 and 2.)

- The first through the seventh vertebrae, called C_1 to C_7, support the head and neck. This is the cervical spine and permits motion in all directions: forward, backward, and rotational.
- The eighth through the nineteenth vertebrae are called T_1 to T_{12} and go down the back of the chest and connect to the ribs. This is the thoracic spine. It helps support the ribs and allows limited body movement in all directions.
- The twentieth through the twenty-fourth, L_1 to L_5, make up the lumbar spine or lower back. These are the source of most back pain. Lumbar vertebrae support the upper part of the body and, like the cervical spine, allow significant motion in all directions.
- The sacrum, the twenty-fifth through the twenty-ninth vertebrae, is referred to as simply S_1. It consists of five fused vertebrae that fit between the pelvic bones and act as the anchor of the spine.
- The coccyx, or tailbone, is the last three fused vertebrae (the thirtieth through the thirty-second) at the bottom of the sacrum. (Very rarely, a person is born with an additional fused vertebrae in the coccyx.)

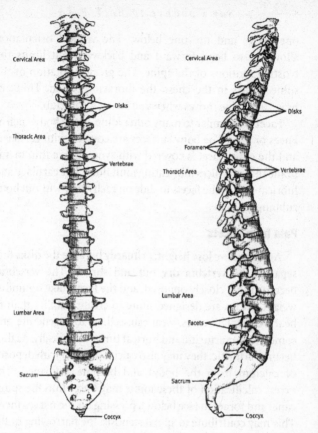

FIGURE 1. *Left:* Front view of spine. Cervical area C_1 to C_7. Thoracic area T_1 to T_{12}. Lumbar area L_1 to L_5. Sacrum S_1. FIGURE 2. *Right:* Side view of spine.

SPINAL JOINTS: FACETS

A system of interlocking small joints, called facets (fah-CETTES) located on the side of each vertebrae, prevent us from turning our heads all the way around like the girl in *The Exorcist*. Each vertebra has four facets that hold it to the one above and the one below. The vertical orientation allows us to bend forward and backward but limits the twisting motions of the spine. The greatest rotation of the spine occurs in the chest, the thoracic portion. Think of how your spine moves when you swing a golf club.

Facets are similar to many other joints in the body, such as knees or hips. The bony surfaces are covered with cartilage, and the entire facet is covered with synovium, a thin membrane that produces lubricating joint fluid. The cartilage and lubricant allow the facets to slide on each other without bone rubbing on bone.

Pain from Facets

As we age, we lose height, primarily because the disks that separate the vertebra dry out and shrink. The vertebrae become more closely opposed, and the facets take on undue weight. Facets are designed more to create stability than to bear weight. This excess wear causes them to degenerate, and some become arthritic and hurt, at times chronically. As they become arthritic, they may also calcify (harden with deposits of calcium from the body) and become deformed. The excess calcification of these joints may bulge into the spinal canal and foramen (see below), pressing on the nerves there. This may contribute to spinal stenosis, the narrowing of the spinal canal. (See Chapter 12.)

SPINAL DISKS

Disks are also joints, but unlike facets, they have no synovium or lubricating fluid. The twenty-three disks between each of the vertebrae work like universal joints, allowing motion in a number of directions. If the vertebrae were in direct contact with each other, the range of motion would be severely limited. Disks play an important role in the gradual process of spinal degeneration, pain, and disability. These semiflexible shock absorbers resemble checker pieces with a leatherlike covering, called the annulus. They are filled with a firm gel-like substance, called the nucleus.

A disk's cushioning ability depends upon how well the gel remains filled with water. At birth, about 90 percent of the gel is water, but by the time we are thirty, the nucleus and annulus have begun to desiccate and become brittle. They crack and fissure. This degeneration results in the disks losing height, the vertebrae coming closer together and slightly wiggling over one another, and our height diminishing. The annulus may tear, allowing disk material to protrude through and press on a nerve root. This may cause pain, weakness, and numbness.

It is the degeneration of the disks that ultimately results in a series of changes of the spinal structures, varying degrees of spinal instability, and the compensatory thickening of the ligaments that support the spine. Later in life, the disk protrusion and thickened ligaments result in spinal stenosis. Significant disk degeneration, especially in the young, may also contribute to spinal instability and cause pain and disability.

Pain from Disks

Discogenic pain comes from a tear in the annulus, with no disk material oozing out onto a spinal nerve. This kind of pain usually is described as deeper than facet pain, but the two frequently coexist. Disks are deeper in the spinal structure than the facets and pain from them cannot easily be provoked by poking the area around the spine. Both facet and discogenic pain may be one-sided but often affect both sides of the back.

Lumbar-disk-related pain (either discogenic pain or pain from disk herniation) is usually worse during the day. It may exist at night and impair sleep. Many postures and activities make it worse: standing, walking, sitting, rising from a bent position, and bending down. Less commonly, lying in bed, with the spine curving into the mattress, may irritate the torn disk or a lumbar nerve compromised by a herniated disk. Anything that puts vertical or bending-related stress on a degenerated, painful disk may worsen the pain.

Cervical-disk-related pain is worse at night because you often turn your head while you sleep. It may also cause pain during the day when you turn your head to look around. When your head bounces around on your neck, such as when you are riding in a car over a rough road, it may also cause pain if you have cervical disk problems.

Thoracic-disk-related pain is rare. When it does occur, it may cause pain in the back or even travel partway around the chest along a rib. Thoracic disk herniation sometimes results in pain that may be confused with other ailments, like heart disease or reflux of the esophagus.

THE SACRUM AND COCCYX

The sacrum is a large triangular bone formed by five fused vertebrae wedged between the pelvic bones. It contains the end of the spinal canal and therefore nerves. The coccyx, or tailbone, consists of three or four tiny fused vertebrae located between the cheeks of the buttocks. It is well padded, so is difficult to fracture.

Right and left sacroiliac joints are formed between the sacrum and the iliac bones of the pelvis which attach to the upper leg at the hip. The sacroiliac joints are not mobile like knees or elbows. If they are injured or degenerate, they cause pain at either side of the upper buttocks. Sometimes sacroiliac-joint pain travels down the leg.

Spinal facets and disks are not differentiated by sex. However, the sacrum is tailored differently for each sex. In men, more of the sacrum is attached to the ilium (part of the pelvis); in women, the sacroiliac joints widen during childbirth. These differences also affect how we walk. The male hip structure tends to be stable during normal walking while women have a natural swaying of the hips when they walk.

Pain at the End of the Spine

The sacrum itself is rarely a cause of pain unless it is fractured or its connection to the lumbar spine is altered. In people with normal bones, sacral fracture may occur from a severe fall. People with severe osteoporosis can fracture the sacrum even from minor trauma. Various types of sacral tumors can cause local pain and damage to the nearby nerves that control bowel, bladder, and sexual function.

Pain in the area of the sacrum also occurs after fusion surgery in which the lumbar spine is surgically fused to the sacrum at L_5–S_1. Sacral pain following this type of fusion is perhaps the most common cause of severe chronic sacral pain in the noncancer patient population. Occasionally, sacral pain is due to sore or tight muscles. It may exist while walking, standing, or sitting.

Chronic, severe tailbone—coccyx—pain is rare. This is fortunate, since it is often difficult to treat. Most people with such pain—coccydynia—complain of pain in the tailbone while sitting. It usually develops following a fall on their rear end, usually squarely backward, as on an icy sidewalk. The tailbone can also be invaded by tumors, which cause pain and often bowel dysfunction.

THE SPINAL CORD AND SPINAL CANAL

The spinal cord is like a fiberoptic cable of nerves, about the thickness of your finger, that carry messages up and down the cord to and from the brain. The cord rests in the hollow space formed by the vertebral arches. This space is the spinal canal. (See figures 3 and 4.)

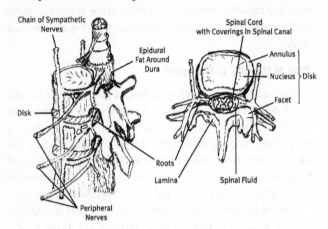

FIGURE 3. Side view of cervical or thoracic spine and top view of cervical spine.

As the principal collection of nervous tissue in the spinal canal, the spinal cord constantly sends messages from the brain to various parts of the body and back. Moving your finger voluntarily, for example, begins with electrical signals that are relayed from your brain down the motor nerve column of your spinal cord to a nerve root and peripheral nerve and into the muscle in your lower arm that lifts your finger. Signals from sensory nerves in your finger go back up the same nerve through a different sensory column in your spinal cord and report to your brain that the job has been accomplished. Reflexive involuntary reactions, such as lifting your finger from a hot stove, are carried out at the level of the spinal cord well before pain signals reach your brain and cause you to say "ouch" and consciously react to the burn.

This exceedingly complex, interconnected system of nerve signals that spreads widely throughout the body often makes it hard to find the exact source of pain. Pain that travels from its source is either radicular or referred pain. Disk pressure on the L_5–S_1 root causes sciatica, pain radiating down the leg because of the compression. This is an example of radicular pain. People are often surprised that the spine is actually the source of pain, numbness, or weakness in their foot. Referred pain mimics radicular pain but is not caused by irritation of a nerve root. Painful lower lumbar facets or a painful sacroiliac joint may also produce sciatica, but this is referred pain. Now you begin to see why diagnosis of painful spinal conditions is often quite complicated.

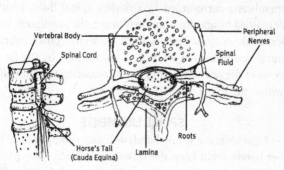

FIGURE 4. Side view of lumbar spine and top view of lumbar spine.

The spinal roots leave the spinal canal, in thirty-one pairs, through the foramen (for-AY-men) which are like little windows on each side of each vertebra, from the neck to the bottom of the sacrum. Once they exit the foramen, these roots are called peripheral nerves (in the periphery or body, outside the spine). These nerves combine with nerves emanating from other foramen, in at times a very complex web of connections. They branch off to supply other parts of the body.

If the spinal cord or a nerve root is severely compressed near the spinal canal, the reflexes associated with that nerve may not work. This reflex loss may be experienced by people with spinal problems who demonstrate lost or diminished reflexes when the doctor taps the appropriate area of the body with a hammer. If certain roots are damaged, your leg will not kick reflexively when your knee is hit, for example.

Spinal Wrap

The brain, spinal cord, and individual roots of the cauda equina (Latin for horse's tail), the place where the spinal roots exit the spinal cord, are wrapped in several layers of protective covering. Closest to the nerves is an ultrathin membrane surrounded by colorless spinal fluid, which is contained by another thin membrane, the arachnoid, which looks like a spiderweb. A thick protective outer layer, the dura, completes the wrap. It is surrounded by the fat and veins of the epidural (Latin for surrounding the dura) space within the spinal canal. (See figure 3.)

SPINAL LIGAMENTS

Ligaments are strong bands of tissue—like powerful rubber bands—that keep the vertebrae in place. They provide stability and restrain excessive movement of the spine. They act like a girdle closely attached to the outside surfaces of the bones and disks. Some ligaments are more elastic and move further than others. Women, for example, have more elastic ligaments connecting the pelvic bones as part of the mechanism to accommodate childbirth. In both sexes, these structures lose elasticity and become stiff with age, which is one reason we lose motion. As we age, ligaments calcify and harden, and some thicken, including those in the spinal canal. They may also become weak.

Several ligaments, outside and inside the spine, make up the spinal support system. There are two big ligaments attached to the outside surfaces of the vertebrae, one in front of the vertebral bodies and disks and one attached to the spinous process: the pointed structures on the back of the vertebrae that make up the bumpy row of bones seen under the skin, along the midline of the back. Another set of ligaments attaches parts of the sides of the vertebrae one to another. There are three ligaments in the spinal canal, the space within the vertebrae in which the spinal cord, cauda equina, and roots reside.

- **Posterior longitudinal ligament (PLL).** From head to pelvis, the back of the vertebral bodies and interspersed disks and the front surface of the spinal canal are covered by the posterior longitudinal ligament (PLL). As the PLL passes down the spine it becomes narrower. By the time it reaches the lumbar spine, this ligament is half its original width and its ability to support the spine and help prevent disk herniations has diminished. This may contribute to the increased likelihood of disk herniations and spinal instability in the lumbar area, the lower back.
- **A pair of ligamenta flava**—or yellow ligaments— line the back of the spinal canal, one on each side. Unlike the PLL, these ligaments do not extend from the top of the entire canal to the bottom. Instead, each pair is located at the connection between two adjacent vertebral bodies, one above and one below.

As disks degenerate, the spine becomes slightly unstable: One vertebral body wiggles a bit over another one, separated by a shrinking, often bulging disk. Compensating for this, some of the supporting ligaments—the ligamenta flava and sometimes the PLL—thicken, just as muscles that perform a lot of work thicken. Eventually, these thickened ligaments bulge significantly into the spinal canal and foramen. The situation is worsened at times by facets that calcify as we age along with ligaments and bulging disks that also take up space in the canal or foramen. These changes may narrow the spinal canal and the foramen, thus squeezing the nerves. This is spinal stenosis (see Chapter 12).

Weakening of the intraspinal ligaments can contribute to spinal instability, called spondylolisthesis (covered in Chapter 11), with resultant slippage of one vertebra over another. Scoliosis, or the development of a crooked spine, can also result from such changes.

Disk herniations, stenosis, spondylosis, and scoliosis—they may coexist with each other—may result in pressure on the spinal cord, the cauda equina, and the nerve roots leaving the spine and supplying the arms, legs, and muscles of the thoracic (rib cage) area. This pressure may result in pain, weakness, and numbness.

The problems from calcification of the PLL are more likely to be evident in the neck, where the ligament is thickest and the diameter of the spinal canal smallest. Asians suffer more frequently from cervical stenosis from calcification of this ligament than members of other ethnic groups.

BACK MUSCLES

You would think that with such a big area to support, our back muscles would be as strong as those of Hercules. Unfortunately, they are not. They play an essential role in the movement of the spine as well as in maintaining normal posture. Most back pain is muscular (see Chapter 6) and improves with time, rest, and, at most, conservative treatment.

There are two very large back muscles:

- The trapezius connects the back of the lower skull to the lowest thoracic vertebra (T_{12}, where the ribs end) and spreads out around the upper back as far as the shoulders. It raises the shoulder and moves the head from side to side and backward.
- The latissimus dorsi, or "lats," as trainers call it, extends from the back of the pelvis to the midthoracic spine and the upper arms. It draws the shoulders down and rotates the arms inward.

Smaller muscles allow the spine to bend to the side or twist around. Part of the psoas muscle connects the front of the spine to the inside of the back of the pelvis. That muscle and the abdominal muscles bend the spine forward, and the latter also push the abdominal organs against the front of the spine, thereby lending it support. (Notice how easy it is to stand up straight when you suck in your gut.) Muscles on either side of and overlying the spine help move the spine backward. If any of these muscles are stiff, normal motion of the spine is limited. This may then result in back pain.

All the muscles are covered with fascia, a membrane that resembles plastic wrap. This enclosure holds the muscle together. The muscle and overlying wrap may cause myofascial pain. This is by far the most common source of back pain.

SPINAL WEAR AND TEAR AND BACK PAIN

The spine wears out from stress. The lumbar spine (lower back) supports the most weight and is the most common area for spine-related pain. The area of greatest spinal degeneration is the lower lumbar spine, attached to the fixed pelvis. The lower cervical spine, just above the shoulders, is the second most likely area to degenerate over time. Consequently, the lumbar and cervical areas have the greatest propensity for disk herniations. (The thoracic spine is least likely to cause chronic pain.)

The vertebrae themselves may cause pain if fractured by day-to-day trauma, suffer an osteoporotic collapse, are weakened by a blood vessel malformation, or invaded by a tumor. If a piece of fractured vertebra presses on the nerves in the spine or spinal cord, serious, possibly permanent pain, weakness, and numbness or bowel, bladder, and sexual disturbance may result.

Another problem occasionally seen is a birth defect involving a hole in the bone in the back of the L_5 vertebra that disconnects the stabilizing facet joint on the side of the defect from the rest of the vertebrae. Over time, this may destabilize the spine, allowing slippage. This type of defect is called spondylolysis (spon-dee-lo-LYSIS). Spondylolisthesis (spon-dee-lo-lies-THEESIS) occurs when a vertebral body slips out of place with respect to the one above or below it, causing spinal instability. Think of that gooseneck lamp with each spinal segment analogous to a ring of the neck. In spondylolisthesis, a ring of the gooseneck lamp is no longer in line with the others. This may result in narrowing of the spinal canal and foramen underlying the area of slippage, resulting in pressure on the nerve roots there. This pressure may become a source of chronic pain, weakness, and numbness unless the spinal instability is surgically corrected.

Can We Slow the Wear and Tear?

Common sense prompts the obvious question: Can the degeneration of disks, facets, ligaments, and other parts of the spine be prevented or at least slowed? It's possible to an extent. Disk degeneration has a genetic basis, about which we can do nothing. Chronic obesity—an epidemic in our society—does place undue stress on the lower spine, including the disks. As for the other parts of the spine and the spine as a whole, you can prevent a good deal of degeneration and pain by treating it with respect. See the last chapter for ways to protect your spine and avoid back pain.

MEDICAL CAUSES OF BACK PAIN

Most back pain results from mechanical disorders of the spine, but, based on my experience, 10 percent to 15 percent of back pain is from medical problems, such as osteoporosis or a cancerous tumor destroying a vertebra. A person with cancer may develop pain from a lymph node (a swollen gland) or tumor pressing on a spinal nerve root. Kidney stones also cause back pain. Usually, it is not possible to determine the cause of such pain based on a person's complaints alone. This is why a detailed history, a specialized physical examination, and excellent quality MRIs, CT scans, X-rays, and electrical tests of nerves emanating from the spine may be needed to diagnose the cause or causes of a painful spinal condition (see Chapter 3). A fifty-six-year-old man came to me with a nine-month history of what he thought was muscle pain in his lower back. It turned out he had advanced cancer, which never would have been diagnosed had we not ordered an MRI.

Key Points to Understanding How Your Back Works

- The spine is a mechanical masterpiece with many components that can be damaged by injury or aging.
- The lumbar back is the most common site for spinal pain, followed by the cervical area just above the shoulders.
- Most back pain is muscular and improves with time, rest and, at most, conservative treatment.

- Much spine-related pain can be prevented by some commonsense lifestyle modifications, such as controlling weight.
- Back pain can also be caused by medical diseases, some of them life-threatening.

Chapter 2

Why a Good Diagnosis Is Hard to Find

Most people think of medicine as a science and therefore can't understand why it is so difficult to find out exactly what is physically wrong with them. Medicine *is* a science, but there is also an *art* to medicine, the art of interpreting everything involved in someone's pain. It means asking the right questions, looking for something in the medical history or lifestyle that may lead to symptoms or indicate risk factors. A good doctor must be intelligent, well educated, curious, interested in solving your problem, experienced with the problem in question, and able to think out of the box when necessary. He or she must also be sensitive to your story and able to ask pertinent questions. How long have you had pain? Can you describe it? When and how did it start? What makes it better or worse? The answers to these questions guide a physical examination and determine what diagnostic tests are ordered and the initial diagnosis and treatment. In the limited resources of today's health-care system, such time-consuming consultation is all too rare. Yet if a doctor hasn't enough time to take a history and conduct a meaningful examination, it is unlikely that a proper diagnosis can be made or beneficial treatment prescribed.

Diagnosis tells *what* is wrong—*why* you have pain—and guides treatment to fix it.

Back pain can be elusive and mysterious, and it keeps millions of Americans in physical, often emotional agony. Because it can be hard to find the source of the pain, some doctors blame it on emotional problems. They do this especially with women. The subjective nature of pain makes it a challenge to understand and treat. The inability to verify the presence of pain or objectively measure its severity leads to an insufficient understanding and treatment of pain and to widespread complaints.

THE COMPLICATIONS OF CHRONIC BACK PAIN

Back pain may be short-lived (acute) or long-lived (chronic), or it may be chronic with acute flare-ups. Acute pain is usually localized and lasts a few hours to a few days. Acute pain usually has an identifiable cause and may result in wincing, screaming, increased sweating, and elevated blood pressure. Acute pain is perceived in the sudden onset of severe muscle spasm in the lower back. You bent over to push that boulder in the garden. As you applied force to it, something snapped in your right lower back, producing excruciating local pain or, worse, when it snapped, a searing pain also shot down your right leg. If this problem lasts over six weeks, it may be deemed chronic.

Chronic pain is often more diffuse than acute pain and usually extends well beyond the original painful site. After a few days, certainly after a few weeks, of living with the severe right lumbar and leg pain in this example, the entire back—both sides—suffers from spasmodic, muscular pain superimposed on the original problem. You feel tight from your lower back to the shoulder blades.

People with a disk herniation in the neck have neck and

arm pain, the arm version of sciatica. They often don't use the arm to which the pain radiates, as this exacerbates it. Over a week, the shoulder becomes stiff and difficult to move: it becomes frozen. This new problem can be as painful as the initial pain from the neck to the arm, often continuing after the neck problem is successfully treated. Without knowledge of the relationship between a frozen shoulder and disk-herniation-related neck and arm pain, the source of the shoulder pain may be misconstrued as being in the neck. In short, we cannot always *easily* find the source of the pain. That doesn't mean that with appropriate effort we can't find it.

If you've suffered from chronic back pain for years, perhaps from the painful aftereffects of a previous back problem that was never adequately treated, you become hypersensitive to relatively innocuous stimuli. If someone touches your arm, say, to put in an IV needle, it may be painful. Unlike your painful back, there is nothing wrong with your arm. In many people with chronic pain, the pain-processing part of their nervous system becomes sensitized. It processes sensory impulses differently. Once this process starts, it is difficult, often impossible, to reverse the sensitization. Often, people simply become increasingly sensitive to mild stimuli, such as a moderate pressure. Fibromyalgia is an example of a disorder of sensitization. Sensitized patients may even develop total body pain in some circumstances: everything hurts from the slightest stimulus. Sadly, sensitized patients are perceived as crazy or attention-seeking by those close to them and, unfortunately, by physicians and other medical personnel unfamiliar with complicated pain problems.

Men and Women Feel Pain Differently

Women seem to have a lower threshold for perceiving pain and a lower pain tolerance than men do. Also, women's coping patterns differ from those of men. Women are often taken less seriously in pain clinics than men. It is often assumed that women in pain have more of a psychological problem than a physical one—even when the women have a clear physical basis for their pain. As a result, women are given more minor tranquilizers and antidepressants than their male counterparts. Men's pain is more likely to be perceived as real. As a result, they are more likely to receive more opiates and fewer psychiatric drugs than women. Cultural and psychological factors appear to be important influences on pain tolerance as well. On the other hand, there is a growing body of information, based on high-quality studies, suggesting a strong biological—as opposed to cultural—basis for the inequality with which men and women perceive and deal with pain. These factors and also individual biological differences may explain the personal differences in pain tolerance in people of the same sex.

REFERRED PAIN:
THE CAUSE IS NOT ALWAYS
NEAR THE EFFECT

Despite the wondrous nature of this incredibly complex and efficient living computer, our nervous system is not perfect. Pain impulses from several different sites in the body may converge on the same area within the spinal cord, which in turn sends information to the brain. Because of this overlap in the nervous system, we may confuse the source of pain with what is in pain.

At any spinal level, the disks, facets, nerve roots, and structures supplied by the roots at that level all feed pain information into the same level of the spinal cord. For example, the nonpainful and painful sensory information— touch, pinprick, and temperature sensation—from the structures (skin, muscles, eyes, ears, mouth, and bone) of the head and those of the upper spine (facets, disks, roots, and the surrounding muscles) both send pain impulses to the same area of the upper spinal cord.

If the upper spine hurts, the brain may erroneously interpret the pain as originating from the head. A large percentage of patients in chronic-headache clinics have an unrecognized and untreated cervical component of their problem. Many of these patients have cervicogenic headaches, that is, ones that originate in the neck. These are especially common following whiplash-type injuries or fusions in the midcervical spine. In most of these patients, their head pain is actually referred pain from the upper cervical facets of the spine. In some, upper cervical disk or muscle pain is responsible for the headache. Failure to diagnose the origin of the headache, due to a lack of understanding of referred neck pain, and to treat it appropriately condemns the patient to a life spent in headache clinics.

What is commonly referred to as sciatica, low back pain running down the buttock or leg, may come from a herniated lower lumbar disk (which can be detected by an MRI) causing nerve pain. True, this may be associated with weakness or numbness, but it is often only a pain complaint. This same kind of pain may represent referred pain from a lower lumbar disk that has degenerated (discogenic pain) but has not herniated. It can also be referred pain, such as muscular spasm of the buttock, a painful sacroiliac joint, of painful lower lumbar facets, that won't be revealed by an MRI.

This is the same mechanism that leads to left arm and shoulder pain during a heart attack. Many people, even physicians, die each year of heart attacks because the pain of the heart is not felt in the chest but is referred to the left arm: patients feel they have a problem with the shoulder or arm and ignore it instead of realizing that their heart is referring the pain from a lack of blood supply. A fatal heart attack may ensue. The nerves that bring pain impulses from the heart enter the spinal cord at the same location as those from part of the left arm. Similarly, women with menstrual cramps may feel the pain over their kidneys, because the nerves supplying the uterus enter the cord at the same level as nerves supplying the area around the kidneys.

High-quality radiological studies, combined with a good history of the pain and a physical examination, may pinpoint the problem. However, at times an MRI or CT scan will not explain the source of the pain. It can be difficult to identify which of these structures is generating the pain, but it is not impossible. Knowledge of patterns of pain referred from various structures aids the physician in suggesting diagnoses that may not otherwise be obtained by other means.

Proper diagnosis is the most critical part of any pain-reduction therapy. The target in the spine must be identified and neutralized for the pain to resolve. It is equally important to understand that if after extensive evaluations by various professionals—don't ever stop at one—no correctable cause for the pain is found, it may be possible to relieve the pain with ongoing medication or other therapies.

TEST-NEGATIVE PAIN:
WHEN THE CAUSE CAN'T BE SEEN

Test-negative pain is pain caused by a problem that cannot be determined using medical technology or expertise. Without blood tests or X-rays and other diagnostic imaging techniques, physicians of past centuries were able to measure very little. They had to rely on patient histories and physical examinations confined to the exterior of the body. Yet the extensive descriptions of disease indicate that they clearly believed in what they could not yet see, touch, or measure.

Headache is one of the most common forms of test-negative pain; most headaches are not due to brain tumors, increased pressure, or infections or bleeding inside the head. The vast majority of headache patients have totally normal brain MRIs, and often any abnormalities that are seen don't explain their headaches. And as you all know, you can't prove or disprove whether someone has a headache by looking at him. You must take his word for it, and society and the medical profession generally accepts a patient's description of headache as proof of headache.

The same should apply to test-negative back conditions but often doesn't. It is often assumed that a patient with back pain whose radiological and physical diagnostic evaluation is negative, is a fake or emotionally disturbed.

Test-negative conditions of the back include:

- most muscle-related or myofascial pain
- pain coming from the facets or joints supporting the spine
- possibly pain due to diseased but not obviously herniated disks

When not adequately treated in a timely fashion, people with test-negative pain may develop significant secondary psychiatric symptoms. Physicians poorly schooled in the intricacies of the appropriate diagnosis and treatment of test-negative painful conditions may help drive some patients with chronic pain to despair.

In many cases, the origin of test-negative pain—pain without a clear-cut anatomical basis, as seen on MRIs or other tests—is difficult to determine without considerable experience and knowledge of patterns of referred pain.

The Importance of Your Story

The history you provide to your doctor is the most important part of the diagnostic process. The more complete and detailed the information, the greater its value. Past and current illnesses are of great importance. For example, a history of cancer may be significant if you have new back pain. An injury, such as from slipping and falling on ice, may have something to do with the development of a herniated disk months later. If you are diabetic, your pain, weakness, or numbness could be due to a form of neuropathy (peripheral nerve damage) as opposed to radiculopathy (a damaged root). Inflammatory arthritis of the spine and its resulting pain is often associated with psoriasis and inflammatory bowel disease. (See Chapter 15.)

Write things down before your visit and organize how you will describe your symptoms. List questions you want to ask. By carefully thinking about your back pain, you will have organized the information necessary to start the diagnostic process. Also, list your medicines and the names and addresses of your other health-care providers.

Here are some questions you should be prepared to answer:

How and When Did the Pain Begin?

Acute back pain is often associated with a specific episode of trauma, such as lifting a heavy bag of groceries from the back seat of your car. Acute pain from minor trauma, especially of a muscular nature—lifting that boulder in your garden over the weekend—often improves with time as the injured spine and surrounding muscles heal. Even pain from an acute disk herniation in the neck or lower back gradually improves without surgery in 70 percent to 80 percent of patients. Systemic illnesses, on the other hand, cause pain that comes on gradually. People with inflammatory arthritis of the spine (spondyloarthropathy) may have had back stiffness and pain for six months or longer when first evaluated for their spinal symptoms. The chronic pain of stenosis usually begins slowly and progresses.

Where Is It Located, and Do You Feel It Anywhere Else?

Low-back pain frequently starts on one side of the spine and quickly spreads to both sides of the spine just above the buttocks. Pain can move from side to side or up and down the leg. Most important is where the pain started and its location most distant from this initial point. I always ask patients with low-back pain if it radiates down their legs and where it terminates. Back pain terminating in the foot is usually due to nerve root pain, especially if there is tingling, numbness, or weakness: clear indications of nerve dysfunction. On the other hand, low aching back pain that radiates down the back of the thigh to the knee—not below—or to the side of the thigh or the groin and is unaccompanied by the symptoms of nerve injury mentioned above is often associated with painful facets. Lumbar discogenic pain frequently causes deep, midline low back pain and occasionally may also radiate down the leg but almost never to the foot. Similar distinctions exist in the neck, helping to distinguish among pain from disk herniation, facets, and painful, nonherniated disks (discogenic pain). Obviously, the physician's initial suggestions from the patient's history must be refined or discarded after the physical examination, radiological tests, and laboratory findings.

How Long Does the Pain Last, and Does It Recur?

This is relevant only for pain that is episodic or fluctuates. When back pain is caused by a muscle spasm, it usually goes away in a few days. However, if it recurs, the pain may last longer and develop into a chronic myofascial pain disorder. If a small, chronically herniated disk presses on an exiting root, neck pain and arm nerve pain may occur from carrying heavy objects, such as carrying luggage when traveling. Fortunately this pain often goes away when the weight-bearing activity ceases unless the disk herniates further. With back pain from medical causes, the important characteristic is duration rather than frequency. Medical back pain—such as that from cancerous tumors that have damaged the spine—is more persistent and may last for years.

What Makes It Feel Better or Worse? When Does It Occur?

If you have a lumbar-facet-related pain, you feel more pain when sitting. When you stand, bending slightly forward reduces pressure on the facets, causing less pain. Facet-related pain is usually vastly reduced when you are in bed. A painful sacroiliac joint and bursa (fluid-filled sac) overlying the hip joint often accompanies painful lumbar facets on one side. While facet pain is less in bed, the pain from the sacroiliac joint and bursa increases there and may disturb your sleep when you lie on the affected side. Sitting, which increases facet pain, may reduce sacroiliac- and bursa-related pain. Neck pain from painful facets or a herniated disk often disturbs sleep. Tossing and turning and entering and leaving dream sleep is hard on a painful neck. Also, sleeping on your side or with your neck arched backward puts increased pressure on the cervical facets and roots compressed by herniated disks. Neck pain may also flare up during the daytime if you turn your head, such as when you parallel-park or change lanes while driving in traffic.

Pain shooting down your arm or leg when you do heavy lifting, cough, or have a bowel movement is usually due to a disk herniation. All of these exacerbating activities increase the pressure in the disk and may force more nuclear disk material to herniate through the torn annulus. This in turn causes more pressure on the root and more radicular pain. Severe disk herniations may cause pain all the time; it is only somewhat less when you are in bed. Pain from cancerous tumors invading the epidural space may actually be worse in bed, from pressure of the tumor on the nerve roots while you are lying down. Medical causes of back pain are more complicated. Degenerative osteoarthritis and also inflammatory arthritis, for example, may hurt more when you are not moving than when you are bending and stretching.

Describe the Quality and Intensity of the Pain

My patients have very precise ways of describing their pain to me. Some perceive their pain in horrifying, vivid terms, like being ripped up by a pack of guard dogs. To others, it may appear to be an act of torture, pain deliberately inflicted, like the slow drip, drip of water on the back of the neck until it seems like a sledgehammer. When someone tells me, "It feels like I've been kicked in the back by a horse," I know he is in pain, whether or not actual bodily damage is occurring. This descriptive ability has a very real foundation in the mysterious way our bodies and brains monitor pain.

When a nerve is compressed it sends a sharp, shooting, burning, or aching pain along the nerve, as in sciatica. Facet-related pain is almost never burning; it usually aches for hours during the day, fluctuating with body position. Kidney stones cause a recurrent gripping back pain that rises quickly to its greatest intensity in twenty to thirty seconds, lasts one to two minutes, and then quickly ceases. It has nothing to do with the position of your body and doesn't lessen when you're in bed.

Does Anyone in Your Family Have the Same Condition?

The genetic basis for disk herniations is just beginning to be explored, with some positive results. It will be many years before we can alter someone's genetic makeup to change the course of their lives in terms of health and disease, not to mention whether we should do it and to whom and who should pay for it. However, a strong family history of spinal disorder may increase your risk of spinal disorders and affect the way you react to pain. If you grew up with a close relative who had significant chronic pain, you may react to pain differently from someone who never had such an experience. Inflammatory arthritis of the spine (spondyloarthropathy) has a genetic predisposition; a test can determine if you are at risk. (See Chapter 15.)

How Does Your Work or Lifestyle Affect It?

This is certainly a loaded question in a country where the majority of people are overweight thus putting added stress on their spines. Most are also more sedentary than not. If you sit all day at a computer, you may develop low back pain—we were not designed to sit all day. Some jobs, sports, or leisure activities may be causing or adding to your back pain. Punctuating your sedentary existence with athletically active weekends—becoming a weekend warrior—is a sure prescription for developing a host of painful disorders or a fatal heart attack.

THE INITIAL PHYSICAL EXAMINATION

Once the doctor has your pain, medical, and family history, the physical examination of your back is next on the agenda.

A clinical examination of your spine should be done

while you are standing, sitting, lying on your back, and on your stomach, so the doctor can see any abnormalities. For example, if either shoulder is elevated or the pelvis is tilted, scoliosis may be indicated (curvature of the spine); this is best discovered when standing. From the side, the doctor can see an increased hunched appearance of the upper spine (kyphosis). Characteristics of poor posture are also best seen from the side. For example, the weight of a protruding abdomen forces your lower back to curve forward.

By applying varying degrees of pressure to your back, a doctor can detect increased muscle contraction or spasm. When back muscles are at rest, they are soft and pliable. Muscles in spasm are tense and firm to the touch and often hurt. The doctor will look for symmetry of muscle contraction in order to locate focal spasm from irritation or injury to muscle or structures underlying them (roots, disks, facets, vertebrae, other muscles) or actual loss of muscle mass from nerve root injury. When the patient is standing at rest, spasm on one side of the lumbar spine may be detected while the other side of the spine is normal.

Gait

Looking at how someone stands and walks yields a tremendous amount of information about his power, sensation, balance, and even mental state. Patients with lumbar stenosis, or narrowing of the spinal canal, prefer to stand and walk bent over, a position that opens the tight canal and relieves their pain. Bending over also reduces pressure on painful facets, so people with lumbar-facet-related pain may walk and stand in a slightly bent fashion. The stance of people with lumbar-disk herniations can suggest to the experienced physician whether a disk is herniated centrally into the canal or to the side, into the foramen. A person with a lumbar-disk herniation to one side of the spine—in the foramen—tends to lean away from the painful side, thus drawing the root away from the disk herniation and alleviating pressure on the root and pain. One having lumbar-disk herniation more toward the midline, in the canal, leans toward the side of the herniation, thus reducing the stretch on the root caused by the disk herniation.

Examining gait permits evaluation of the entire nervous system, from the feet to the brain. For example, a limp suggests weakness or pain in the lower back or leg. It may also imply significant numbness. If chronic, a limp may cause pain elsewhere. People who limp from a one-sided problem often develop secondary pain from their lopsided gait. It may cause one-sided pain in a lower lumbar facet or the sacroiliac joint. It may cause myofascial pain in the buttock, thigh, and groin. Bursitis of the covering of the hip joint can be another result. In other words, it can lead to chronic back and sciatica-like pain from the untreated disk herniation's pressing on a nerve. In some patients like this, even if the disk is successfully treated surgically and the nerve pain goes away, the facet and other pain mentioned above may need treatment as well. (See facet pain and myofascial pain in later chapters.)

If the sole of a patient's shoe is excessively worn down in the toe area, I can tell that he or she is not walking normally. This is confirmed by watching the patient walk. He or she has what we call a dropped foot: muscles that pick up the toes from the floor are not working properly, usually because of damage to the L_5 spinal root or the sciatic nerve in the buttock or leg.

A gait suggestive of excessively tight muscle in both legs is a phenomenon called spasticity and results from damage to the brain or spinal cord. It can affect the arms or legs. It is often seen after a severe stroke, multiple sclerosis, or in conjunction with cerebral palsy.

Range of Motion

Range of motion tests tell us a great deal. An injured lumbar spine will have limited normal motion because the muscles tightened to protect it. If injury to the spine is one-sided, the spine is tilted to the side of the shortened muscles in spasm. If you have difficulty straightening your legs, it may be from tightness of the buttocks and the hamstring muscles in back of the thighs. When you bend forward then return to an upright position, the motion and pain it may induce can reveal information about the injured structures that cause it.

When bending to one side, you stretch the muscles on the opposite side of your spine and compress the facets on the side to which you bend. Pain on the *same* side as the bending suggests pain emanating from the facet joints on that side; a stretching sensation with pain on the *opposite* side from the bending suggests a muscle injury with spasm.

People with lumbar discogenic pain often arise from a bent position in a ratchetlike fashion. Because of increased pain, those with facet pain and stenosis may not be able to arch their lumbar spines backward. Cervical-facet pain makes it difficult to arch your neck or bend it. These maneuvers increase pressure on the cervical facets, worsening the pain. Those with lumbar disk herniations may have difficulty bending to one side or the other, depending on the location of the herniation.

If you have one-sided cervical radicular pain (from a disk herniation), you may often move the arm on that side less frequently, because movement hurts. Over time, such restricted arm movement causes the soft tissues around the shoulder to become stiff from lack of use. This in turn results in a frozen shoulder with a reduced range of motion. Attempting to force the arm beyond its acquired limitation—usually by raising it sideways away from your body—results in tremendous shoulder pain. This kind of movement is often so restricted that you can't move your arm so that it is parallel to the floor, much less over your head. Physical therapy can eventually unfreeze the arm. Any examination of a patient with cervical nerve pain should include a range-of-motion evaluation of the arm on the side of the pain.

Testing Power

Your doctor will test the various muscle groups in your limbs in a search for weakness, presumably due to a spinal root's being injured. Many people come to me for pain relief—from stenosis, for example—and are totally unaware of their weakness. They think that they walk a certain way from pain when in fact their limp results from both pain and weakness.

Obviously, treating a patient's pain without addressing and correcting the cause of weakness—usually with decompressive surgery—is not good medicine. Other causes of weakness include damage to other parts of the nervous system: strokes of the brain or spinal cord, arthritic pressure on the cord in the canal, and peripheral neuropathy. These causes may be distinguished from those related to nerve-root damage through physical examination and radiological and electrophysiological tests.

Testing Sensation

While you are seated on the exam table, your legs dangling, the doctor will touch both arms, thorax, abdomen, and legs with a dull object and a sharp one (a clean pin), examining your perceptions of light touches and pinprick. These sensations are often abnormal—either heightened or diminished—in patients with any of a host of neurological problems, including stroke, spinal-cord damage, nerve-root damage, and neuropathy. He or she will also evaluate your ability to discern vibration. This is done by applying a tuning fork to the joints in the fingers and toes and possibly elsewhere in the limbs. Your doctor will also assess your ability to feel what position your joints are in as he bends your toes, fingers, and if needed, feet, lower legs, wrists, and lower arms. Diminished vibratory sense and the inability to determine what position the joints are in—toes and fingers bent up or down, for example—is characteristic of neuropathy or damage to part of the spinal cord or brain.

Testing Reflexes

Hitting the back and front of the elbow, the middle of the forearm, the front of the bottom of the knee, and the back of the ankle with a rubber hammer is another test of reflexes, as mentioned in Chapter 1. An absence of knee reflex, for example, corresponds to an abnormality of the L_3 or L_4 nerve root. On the other hand, quick reflexes may suggest damage to the brain or spinal cord. Diffusely diminished reflexes suggest neuropathy. Other reflexes—retraction of the scrotum when its side is lightly stroked or contraction of the anus when it is lightly stroked—also tell the physician about the integrity of the lower spinal roots and the peripheral nerves supplying these organs.

Control of the bowels, bladder, and sexual function can all be affected by damage to the brain, spinal cord, or cauda equina, the spinal roots coming out of the spinal cord at about L_1. Cord or cauda injury can result from a massive disk herniation or a fractured vertebra; the resultant compression of these vital neurological structures can cause bowel and bladder damage.

Muscle Tone and Appearance

The loss of muscle mass can occur when the nerves that supply them are damaged. This kind of damage can come from long-standing compression of the roots, a chronic disk herniation or stenosis, for example. Damage to the S_1 root can cause calf muscle loss. This is easily seen on physical examination, especially if one side is affected and the other is less so or not at all.

Mechanical Maneuvers

When you are lying flat on your back on the examining table, your doctor may raise your leg up in the air to pull on the roots that supply the sciatic nerve and the nerve itself. Most patients can allow their leg to be raised so it is perpendicular to the floor. The exacerbation of pain shooting from your back or buttock down your leg to the toes while your leg is passively raised suggests disk herniation that affects those roots. Pressure on the roots supplying the nerve or on the nerve itself can cause this response. While you lie on your back, the doctor may bend your knee and rotate your leg outward, pointing your heel toward your groin. This movement tests the integrity of your hip joint: If you have arthritis in the hip, you will feel pain in the hip and possibly the upper thigh, groin, and buttock.

Other Tests

If you have heart disease, stomach ulcers, cancer, or other medical problems, other organ systems need to be evaluated, physically or by laboratory tests, such as a PSA blood test for prostate disease.

The history and physical examination are often all we need to determine the likely cause of back pain so additional tests may be unnecessary. However, the source of much back pain, especially when chronic, is not always easy to find. In the next chapter you will find information about radiological diagnostic tests and what they can and cannot determine.

Key Points in Getting Your Back Pain Correctly Diagnosed

Your pain complaints should be taken seriously and evaluated using the conventional tools, including a good history of the problem, physical examination, and high-quality tests. When this standard evaluation, including radiological, physiological, and other conventional tests, is negative or when what is abnormal on the office evaluation and laboratory tests doesn't fit the pain, you will more likely get a correct diagnosis if the following criteria are met:

- The doctor believes your pain is real
- The doctor believes pain is a personal and subjective experience, colored by personality, personal history, and culture
- The doctor knows the full range of spinal-pain syndromes and their causes
- The doctor takes a full history, making note of medical problems that may contribute to or cause the pain, and focuses on the details of the pain location, type of pain, and what makes it better or worse

- The doctor performs a physical examination, directed at finding the cause of the pain
- The doctor employs, where appropriate, less conventional tests, such as diagnostic nerve blocks (see Chapter 3) or other minimally invasive tests or in some cases, even sophisticated imaging studies to identify the source of the pain and understand how it is processed in the brain.

Chapter 3

Will Pictures Tell the Story? What to Know about Diagnostic Tests

In the absence of some evidence of a serious problem, such as a big disk herniation or cancer, the physician has to wade through a swamp of possible causes of back pain. The spine and potentially painful structures lie buried deep beneath the muscles and skin, so physical examination is not possible.

To properly diagnose painful spinal conditions, nothing less than excellent radiological studies are needed, because doctors must be able to see subtleties in the anatomy. Often, insurance companies don't want to pay for high-quality studies, so you may have to challenge them. If you go to a photographer to have a professional portrait made of your face, you don't want him to take one snap with a throwaway camera and send you out the door. You require even more care from a radiologist who is looking for clues to improve your health and quality of life. The quality and presentation of the films should both be excellent. If a technician needs to sample the area of the anatomy thoroughly, with many images, he or she should cover the whole area in

41

question, not skip some of it, especially not for cost reasons.

Here's why. In many instances, a disk herniates upward toward the nerve root, as it leaves the dura, well before it travels down to enter the foramen. Occasionally it travels downward. In either direction, it moves beyond the area behind the disk space. Disks can also break into pieces, and a free-floating fragment can migrate away from the disk space to irritate a root above it. If an MRI covers only the area through the disk space, the upward extension of the disk or its fragment and the pressure exerted on the nerve root at that location will not be seen. The same applies for older people with arthritic narrowed spines. An arthritic protuberance pressing on a nerve root can be missed by poor MRI sampling of the spine. The diagnosis will also be missed and the treatment misguided and unsuccessful. To save money, many managed-care and public facilities produce MRIs with limited sampling of the spine, running the risk of missing disk fragments pressing on nerve roots, causing pain and possible neurological dysfunction. Physicians treating such patients will often misdiagnose them, either not referring to surgery those who have a surgical problem or, worse, operating on the wrong area of a spine with several abnormalities. It is imperative to relate the patient's complaints and abnormalities of physical examination to the radiological findings.

There are many ways to see inside your back. All have both benefits and limitations. Some doctors favor tests that fit their specialty. And, as mentioned, health insurance may also limit your options.

Always ask your doctor what the tests will determine and if they will find the source of pain. What will they see in the picture? What won't they see? The lack of correlation between clinical symptoms and diagnostic findings is characteristic of the most common causes of back pain. They are test-negative causes.

Based on autopsy findings, by age fifty, nearly all adults show evidence of changes in the spine from aging, including narrowing of the disk space. MRI studies of normal people—those without pain—reveal that approximately two-thirds of them nevertheless have disk abnormalities that may cause it but clearly do not always do so.

Check the reputation of the facility where you are sent for diagnostic tests. Be wary of storefront testing sites unaffiliated with reputable medical centers. Look for medical centers whose radiological and diagnostic testing departments have excellent reputations.

CONVENTIONAL X-RAYS

Plain X-rays are useful in evaluating the appearance of the spine, and they are excellent at showing the spatial arrangement of the vertebrae. They show the distance between vertebrae, which indicates the health of the corresponding disk. Such X-rays also detect changes in bony architecture that may have resulted from prostate or breast cancer or osteoporosis. They reveal such disorders as spinal slippage and scoliosis and allow the measurement of the degree of curvature of the spine that is present in scoliosis.

However, plain X-rays tell us little about the *inside* of the spine, about disk herniations, stenosis, arthritic outgrowths, or calcified structures pressing on the spinal cord or roots causing pain or dysfunction.

In most circumstances, X-rays are not indicated unless you've been in pain for six to eight weeks. Your doctor will order them if there is concern about medical disorders, such as arthritis that affects the facet joints. Also keep in mind that very few physicians—other than experienced radiologists or spine specialists—can accurately interpret an X-ray and relate it to your problem and examination. This is one more reason to seek out the best spine specialist, even for the evaluation of a routine test like this.

Flexion-Extension X-rays

When pain is caused by improper movement of the spine, flexion-extension X-rays can show the spine when it is bent forward (in flexion) and backward (in extension). This shows any slippage occurring between the vertebral bodies during movement. Sometimes similar X-rays should be obtained of the body bending from side to side to detect possible slippage in that direction.

MAGNETIC RESONANCE IMAGING (MRI)

Unlike X-rays, both MRI and CT can see inside the spine, where problems may be, and are the most sensitive tests for identifying the location of a disk herniation and nerve compression.

- MRI is a diagnostic radiological device that provides images of the body through the use of exposure to a magnetic field without the use of radiation.
- X-rays may be entirely reasonable for someone with a herniated disk, but MRI scans identify the size and location of disk herniations, including the migration of extruded disk fragments.
- MRI is superior to CT in detecting soft-tissue injuries, such as tears in the annulus, fat in the epidural space, tumors, and blood-vessel malformations.
- Previous spinal surgery can also be evaluated with MRI. For example, it can detect small residual frag-

ments of disk within the surgical scar that press on nerve roots and cause otherwise unexplained pain.

For patients having an MRI within a year of surgery, an intravenous dye—gadolinium—is injected. This dye is incorporated within scar tissue from previous surgery but not disk fragments, allowing MRI visualization of them.

In some areas, such as where the upper neck and the base of the skull meet, MRIs can be done on the head as it is bent forward then backward on the neck. This may reveal a painful condition caused by abnormal motion of the skull on the cervical spine or compression of the spinal cord or nerve roots by bony abnormalities on the base of the skull and the vertebral bodies, including the joints connecting and the ligaments supporting them. Pain from compression of nervous system structures may be exacerbated by these movements.

If possible, avoid open-air MRIs, because they do not result in the best images. If you are claustrophobic, use an MRI facility with a staff that can take the time to talk you through the procedure, possibly letting you rest outside the scanner between sequences. Using tranquilizers also may be beneficial in getting a claustrophobic patient through a closed MRI.

A stand-up MRI has not been shown to be superior to one taken lying down.

Who Should Not Have an MRI?

An MRI does not expose one to radiation, but it cannot be used if you have metal clips with magnetic properties from surgery in your body. There is a risk that the clips will move or heat up under the influence of the magnet. Modern clips are safe. Metal hardware from spinal-fusion surgery may distort the image. The MRI machine will also short-circuit a pacemaker, with lethal consequences. Some chronic pain patients have devices implanted in the spine to help control their pain. The programming of spinal-cord stimulators and intraspinal drug-infusion pumps may be scrambled by the MRI radio signals. With pumps delivering narcotics and other medications into the spinal fluid, this could result in lethal overdosing or painful underdosing and narcotic withdrawal. Incorrectly programmed stimulators may produce significant pain. In an MRI, the electrodes of the stimulators may heat up over the underlying spinal cord, producing irreversible cord damage. Metallic devices outside the field of view of the MRI—say, a hip replacement in a patient getting a spinal MRI—do not interfere. An MRI takes twenty to thirty minutes, depending on how many studies are undertaken.

COMPUTED AXIAL TOMOGRAPHY (CT)

CT uses a computer to deliver X-rays that are passed through the body at various angles to produce complex images of the internal structure of body organs, including the spine. It provides more detailed information than plain X-rays. This test is appropriate for people who cannot have MRI because of pacemakers, metal clips, or claustrophobia. CT scans are taken while you lie flat on your back in the center of an open circular overhead structure that supports the scanning machine. This test lasts ten to twenty minutes.

- For many clinicians, the bony anatomy is easier to interpret on CT than on MRI.
- CT scans also assess soft tissues, including disks, ligaments, and nerve roots, but not as well as MRIs.
- CT is useful in telling us if spinal fusions are intact

or if there are defects in the vertebrae that could lead
to spinal instability or slippage.

- On CT we can see any small bony disk fragments,
  pieces of arthritic outgrowth, or calcified ligaments
  as well as, if not better than, on MRI.
- CT evaluations of the chest and abdomen are
  superior to MRIs since breathing can alter the
  quality of the MRI but not the CT image.
- Internal metal hardware from previous surgery
  can distort the CT image, too.

MYELOGRAM

The myelogram is a powerful test and is the best study
for evaluating pain in people with complex spinal problems.
Unlike CT scans and MRIs, myelograms permit visualization of the effects of body movement of the spine on the
intraspinal contents.

Radiological dye that can be seen on the myelogram is
instilled under X-ray guidance into the spinal fluid of the
lower or upper spine. With the dye in place, you may be
tilted in various positions or bent forward and backward to
determine the effect of movement on structures, such as the
yellow ligaments, to see if they compress nerves and cause
pain. The dye used for myelography eventually becomes
diluted, so the test must be completed within an hour for
the neck and around two hours for the thoracic and lumbar
spine. Following the injection of the dye, while the dye is
present in the spinal fluid, a CT scan is also obtained, imaging the effect of any root or spinal-cord compression by
disk herniations, calcium deposits, thickened yellow ligaments, or displaced vertebrae. Because of the spinal puncture, you must lie down for several hours following the
myelogram. Resting in these positions reduces the risk of

temporary headaches, which sometimes develop after the test.

Myelograms are being superseded by MRIs and CT scans, but they can still help doctors make or confirm a diagnosis. Myelograms are still the best diagnostic test to evaluate complex spinal problems, especially those existing after previous surgery. For example, they enable the determination of the extent of stenosis (narrowing of the spinal canal) with changes in bodily posture. Stenosis, and the pain and dysfunction from it, is worse with the back bent backward (extended); better with the spine flexed forward. To decide which levels need surgical decompression and which may be left alone, a myelogram with flexion-extension views is still the gold standard.

A CT followed by a myelogram with flexion and extension views is sometimes used for an even more definitive diagnosis. First the myelogram is done in the flexion and extension positions, then the patient is taken to a CT scanner in the same building while the dye from the myelogram is still in place.

DISCOGRAM

Discography can confirm or eliminate disks as potential sources of pain. If MRI shows a tear in the annulus or disk covering, usually coupled with other signs of disk degeneration, a discogram may determine if one or more disks are the cause of pain. Disks that appear completely normal on MRI are almost never the cause of pain, and not all disks that appear abnormal on MRIs cause pain.

Guided by a fluoroscope or a CT scanner, an experienced physician injects radiological dye into the suspicious disk or disks and also into the disk above and below. Mixed with sterile water or local anesthetic, this dye slightly inflates the disk. The normal response is a slight sensation of pressure.

The abnormal response is an unequivocal reproduction of the usual pain. The most important role of discography is to discover which disk is painful. It should never be used as the only test.

ELECTROMYOGRAM (EMG)

Electrodiagnostic tests can help confirm the suspicion of nerve damage from spinal compression of roots as opposed to damage to nerves once they leave the spine. They evaluate peripheral nerves that travel beyond the spinal cord and show abnormalities in both nerve and muscle function. They can help diagnose the following:

- radiculopathy pain from nerve-root irritation;
- peripheral neuropathy, a disorder of the peripheral nerves, commonly seen in diabetics;
- muscle diseases caused by inflammation of the muscles.

However, these tests do not identify the specific cause of the dysfunction. They must be used in conjunction with a history, physical examination, and laboratory and radiological studies.

EMG, which evaluates the electrical activity generated by muscles at rest and at work, is usually combined with a nerve conduction velocity (NCV), which measures the speed of the transmission of the electrical signal along roots and nerves. These tests are carried out by sticking thin needles into the muscles or placing a special device over the nerves to electrically stimulate them and measure the speed of electrical impulses along them. The process is mildly painful. For diagnosing back problems, these tests are most often used to evaluate pain that radiates down an arm or leg.

When nerve roots and peripheral nerves are damaged, some fibers function inadequately. Some may die. The parts of the muscle supplied by damaged or dead nerve fibers behave electrically different from those still supplied by normal fibers. Muscles without their usual nerve supply are easily irritated, a phenomenon that can be measured by the EMG needles. However, when a nerve is injured, the results of the damage may not show up for about three weeks, so if electrodiagnostic tests are performed too early, they will miss the abnormality.

If radiological tests show the cause of the pain, in most painful spinal disorders there is no reason for an EMG. I estimate that 90 percent of EMG studies performed in patients with spinal-related pain are unnecessary.

DIAGNOSTIC NERVE BLOCKS

Nerve blocks are used for diagnosis or when combined with long-acting injected steroids are used as therapy to provide days to months of relief from painful spinal conditions. Local anesthetics are injected around a nerve to block the transmission of various impulses. Different impulses are blocked as the strength of the anesthetic increases. Progressively, blocked first are impulses in the nerves governing blood pressure and flow to an area (sympathetic nerves), followed by impulses controlling sensation (including pain), and finally those that control muscle power.

Chemicals that block this conduction wear off over time as they are broken down by body enzymes. Several things determine how fast they work and how long they last:

- the chemical properties of the anesthetic
- the addition of other drugs to the anesthetic
- site of the injection of the anesthetic (into the

skin, near a peripheral nerve, or into the epidural space as opposed to into the spinal fluid)

Commonly used local anesthetics (occasionally combined with another drug to increase their length of action) used for local skin injections, peripheral nerve blocks, and epidurals include:

- **Lidocaine** (Xylocaine) acts quickly and lasts from about one to three hours
- **Mepivacaine** (Carbocaine), often used by dentists, acts fairly quickly and lasts one and a half to three hours
- **Bupivacaine** (Marcaine) may take longer to begin to work but lasts two to twelve hours. (I never use Marcaine because it can cause cardiac arrest if too much inadvertently gets into the bloodstream.)

When properly chosen and used judiciously, local anesthetics are a godsend in the control of local pain during procedures and for diagnostic blocks (think of having a root canal without local anesthesia). However, there are some risks associated with their use that color which ones are used for evaluation and treatment of chronic pain.

There are cautions to observe with these procedures. Allergic responses to local anesthetics can happen and may be severe. They can effectively be treated medically. Local anesthetics given in high concentrations that get into the bloodstream may have deleterious systemic effects, including seizures and cardiac arrest. If the needle delivering the local anesthetic to the root or epidural space pierces the dura and arachnoid so that the anesthetic gets into the spinal fluid, partial or total spinal anesthesia may occur. This results in a severe temporary fall in blood pressure and possibly the inability to move or breathe. If this happens a physician—usually an anesthesiologist—must artificially restore the patient's blood pressure and respiration until the anesthetic wears off. (In most high-quality pain management, anesthesiologists are usually present.) Remember this when considering epidural steroids (usually given with local anesthetics) as opposed to oral steroids. Epidural steroids are not just a little shot in the back (see Chapter 18).

Diagnostic nerve blocks should be used only to help confirm diagnoses suggested by other means (such as a description of pain, a focused examination, and high-quality radiological studies). By themselves, they are not precise enough to pinpoint a source of pain. In the context of the total evaluation, these blocks may help identify the pain generators—the structures responsible for causing pain.

Unfortunately, the injected chemicals, being liquid, can spill into surrounding areas, even on other nerves. By blocking structures other than the target, the block's precision is reduced. Thus we need to perform blocks using only a small amount of liquid with good radiological guidance. If a block fails to stop pain, the blocked area is not a source or at least not the only source of pain. If the block does temporarily relieve pain, the blocked area *may* be the principal pain-generating structure. Because of these caveats, these blocks should never be used alone as a diagnostic tool.

BONE-DENSITY TESTS

Bone-density tests have become a fairly routine screening device to detect osteoporosis in postmenopausal women. This test measures bone mass. Low bone mass results from a loss of calcium from the bone and leads to increased risk of fracture. The method most used to determine bone mineral density in the spine and the thighbone is dual energy X-ray absorptiometry (DEXA or DPX). Using low-energy X-rays, we can determine the difference in the absorption of the beam by the bone versus that by the soft tissues. The difference in absorption corresponds to the amount of calcium in the bones. Postmenopausal women, andropausal men, and men or women taking cortico-steroids are most likely to develop osteoporosis and are therefore the best candidates for this test.

BONE SCAN

Bone scan (radionuclide imaging) is used to detect frac-tures and such bone abnormalities as arthritis, infections, and metastasized cancer. Some fractures are very small and cannot be detected by plain X-rays. Bone scans are able to identify these fractures regardless of the cause. A small amount of a radioactive material is injected into a vein; a few hours later, the scanning begins. This can take up to an hour. Areas reacting to an injury (fracture or inflammation) show up as a dark or hot spot on the scan. Most bone cells are in a dormant state. The increased activity shown on the scan results from the increased absorption of the radioac-tive material by the bone cells trying to heal the injury. The presence of the hot spot cannot indicate a specific diagnosis: tumors, infections, fractures, and arthritis all cause dark spots on the scans. Additional radiographic evaluation or blood tests are needed to reach a specific diagnosis.

LABORATORY TESTS

If there is reason to believe that the cause of your back pain is a medical condition, blood tests are useful.

A complete blood count (CBC) measures red and white blood cells and platelets. A high white count may be a sign of infection, such as a spinal abscess, which is causing pain. Other tests can determine if inflammation is present.

Chemical tests of the blood and urine measure bone chemistry, liver and kidney function, and hormone levels. Some components of these tests may show abnormal results in people who take drugs, have cancers, and disorders that cause osteoporosis.

Nonsteroidal anti-inflammatory drugs (NSAIDs) are often prescribed to treat back pain. These drugs, though effective, can cause bleeding ulcers, loss of kidney function, and liver inflammation. Those who take these drugs for a long time are given blood tests to monitor the blood and liver and kidney function.

Key Points about Diagnostic Tests

- Always get the best possible radiological and diagnostic tests. Quality varies a great deal. If necessary, pay out of pocket for high-quality radiological tests, especially MRIs and myelograms.
- Ask your doctor what the tests will show and why they are needed.
- The majority of EMGs ordered by doctors for evaluation of spinal problems are unnecessary.
- X-rays cannot image the inside of the spine.
- MRI, CT scans, and myelograms are best at showing the inside of the spine.
- Myelograms are the best diagnostic tests for evaluating the effect of spinal movement on compression of the spinal cord or roots.
- Discograms and nerve blocks can help identify a disk or other structure causing pain but should be used only to confirm a diagnosis gained from a more comprehensive evaluation.

Chapter 4

Finding the Doctor Who Can *Really* Help You

Many of my patients come to me after spending years going from one doctor to another in an endless search for the one who can cure their pain. Myrna had emigrated to this country from Bosnia and came to me with excruciating cramping in one of her legs that had lasted for two years. Ten years before she had had the same problem, and a neurosurgeon in Italy removed a disk herniation in her lower back with excellent results. Myrna returned to work as a housekeeper and had been pain-free for eight years. One night as she was mopping the floor, she felt the pain shoot down from her back and thought it was that same disk acting up again.

After evaluating Myrna with an MRI, her American doctor saw no anatomical explanation for her pain. He prescribed drugs, but they did not relieve it in the slightest. He then referred her to a pain-management specialist, who at first tried more drugs then decided to implant a pump to deliver morphine into her spine, which was an extraordinary step usually used only for extraordinary pain. Even after this high-tech method of pain control, she required additional pain pills. And she was still in so much pain that she could not sit down.

Myrna's son, Joseph, concerned about his mother's painful existence, brought her to see me. She had to lie on a couch when she came to my office. The MRI she brought me was two years old and of low quality, yet I was able to detect what appeared to be a recurrent disk herniation, of the same disk that had caused the original problem, diagnosed and correctly treated in Italy. I wanted a better MRI that would give me a fuller picture, but because of the difficulty in performing an MRI in the presence of an implanted morphine pump and her previous surgery having complicated her anatomy, I decided to send her for a CT scan coupled with a myelogram. These confirmed that she had a small disk herniation in the old location. It had squeezed a nerve root near it, causing her two years of agony.

Myrna should not have been taking long-term pain medication and should not have had the pump. She should have had surgery. Once she had the disk operation, she was fine, especially when the residual effects of the medication disappeared from her system. Interestingly, the surgeon who performed the discectomy noticed that the pump was never properly connected in the first place, another reason she suffered so much for two years.

When I saw the MRI, I thought the problem was a recurrent disk herniation at the same site as the one before. When Myrna bent over to mop the floor and experienced back pain, she recognized her problem. She was absolutely right, but no doctor listened to her. Instead, they put her on a painful, very expensive, inappropriate, and ineffective course of treatment. Her case illustrates the challenges a patient faces in choosing the physician who will help her in the current atmosphere of medical managed care.

SHOPPING FOR A DOCTOR

Most chronic sufferers from moderate-to-severe pain have changed doctors since their pain began; about a third have changed physicians at least three times. The primary reason for the change is still having much pain even after treatment. Many people give up. About 40 percent of those with moderate-to-severe chronic pain no longer consult with doctors for treatment. These unfortunate patients think the doctor cannot help them, that they will have to deal with their pain themselves: grin and bear it. In theory, anyone with back pain should be able to find the proper doctor and treatment. And in fact, it is easier if you know how to shop.

A trusting relationship between doctor and patient is essential. The question is which doctor to trust and how to choose him or her. The inadequate relief of pain results from people's failure to doctor-shop effectively. Often, people insured with HMOs look in their health-care directory and hope for the best. Some are unaware that they can challenge the system and become well-informed patients.

Don't expect your medical insurance company to help you. If you call to ask where you can find a doctor who specializes in neurosurgery, you will be asked, "What's your zip code?" They assume that nobody wants to go far from home to find a doctor. Consult more knowledgeable sources, like doctors you know and other patients. Ask them what hospitals and doctors have the best reputations for treating your kind of back pain. Books like this one may be of help with an approach to doctor-shopping, but they will not give you the names of doctors in any given area. The internet may be consulted *but is no guarantee of quality.* (You have no good way of determining the thoroughness, accuracy, and objectivity of what you read on the internet.) Professional medical associations, like your state medical society, may be consulted, but they are not permitted to tell you that one physician is superior to another. Medical school affiliation usually implies higher-quality care, but this rule may not always hold up for a given individual.

Once your primary-care physician learns that you are willing to go to great lengths to get help, he or she may help you interpret the information you gather. Many of my patients come from various parts of the country; they were sent to me by physicians who reviewed my website at their request.

Linda came to me from the Midwest, where she does sophisticated laboratory work in a highly technological firm. Following lumbar disk surgery several years ago, she continued to experience such significant back and right leg pain that she considered applying for disability. There seemed to be no evidence of anything left in her spine to cause pain from pressure on a nerve root or that the spine was unstable. She had been to several local pain clinics without result, in spite of competent attempts to help her. She was also about to get married and wanted to begin her married life in a positive state. Linda traveled to New York to see me. I was able to help her through two pain-relieving procedures. I lesioned—selectively destroyed—nerves from her lower lumbar facet joints. Also, I partially lesioned a ganglion—a neural computer governing sensation and pain—of the lumbar nerve root that was giving her leg pain. These procedures ended all her pain (something I never really expect to happen).

Linda's fiancé paid for the trip and the costs of her care with his credit card. He even took out another credit card to assure that she would have enough money in the event it was necessary. He gladly took on debt so that she could get proper treatment. She danced at her wedding six months later and was a very happy bride. They both feel the trip to

New York and the financial investment in her care was more than worth it.

Make it your responsibility to choose doctors who have not only a great deal of compassion but also up-to-date knowledge and experience so they can give their patients the best medical care possible.

In all medical areas—especially my specialty of neurology—compassion, patience, dogged determination to resolve a problem, and intelligence and creativity in seeking solutions are absolutely essential to success—and professional and personal satisfaction. I am not the only physician who thinks this way. Find your own. But find one who takes you seriously.

PHYSICIANS WHO TREAT BACK PAIN

There are approximately one hundred thousand licensed physicians in the United States, of which only an estimated four thousand have training in controlling intractable pain. Some of these four thousand may prescribe narcotics for chronic pain, while others may just perform pain-relieving procedures, such as nerve blocks including epidurals, discograms, and lesions of various kinds.

Musculoskeletal back pain (pain originating around the muscles), arthritis, fibromyalgia, and osteoporosis may be best diagnosed and treated by rheumatologists. Physiatrists or physical medicine and rehabilitation specialists also treat musculoskeletal pain. Neurologists, neurosurgeons, and orthopedic surgeons specializing in spinal surgery diagnose and treat more complex back pain, such as that caused by disk herniations, stenosis, and spondylolisthesis.

Anesthesiologists who specialize in the treatment of chronic pain prescribe various kinds of pain medications, including narcotics. They are the most likely to use nerve blocks, epidurals, and other pain-relieving procedures including spinal cord stimulation, implanted pumps, and radiofrequency lesioning techniques for pain control. (See Chapter 18.)

Endocrinologists specialize in hormonal systems and also diagnose and treat osteoporosis.

Neurologists diagnose and medically treat problems of the nervous system, for example peripheral neuropathy, strokes, and multiple sclerosis, all of which can cause severe chronic pain. Regrettably, not all are adept in treating complicated patients with chronic pain of spinal origin. Many are not well trained in the use of narcotics to control severe pain. However, some—those with a special interest in the treatment of chronic pain—have greater expertise than other medical specialists in diagnosing and treating pain emanating from peripheral nerves, the spine, or damaged brain or spinal cord. They are perhaps better than most physiatrists at diagnosing and treating nerve-related pain. However, pain of musculoskeletal origin, for which there is no radiological diagnostic basis, may be better recognized by physiatrists than neurologists. As a rule, neurologists use only medication in therapy; they do not perform pain-relieving procedures, though there are exceptions, myself included.

Neurosurgeons specialize in the surgery of the nervous system, including the spine. They may perform various types of spinal operations, including fusions, depending on their training. Some may use radiofrequency procedures on certain nerves in or leading to or from the spine. They are usually the only specialists who perform procedures to selectively destroy pain pathways in the brain and spinal cord. Some may also implant spinal cord and brain stimulators and drug pumps. Some are more likely to recommend spinal surgery than the more conservative neurologists or other medical specialists, a recommendation that is not always incorrect.

Oncologists treat cancer. Cancer-related back pain is best diagnosed and treated by them or by neurologists, anesthesiologists, and neurosurgeons with expertise and training in cancer.

Orthopedic surgeons specialize in the surgery of the skeletal system. Some specialize in surgical treatment of spinal disorders. They may be more likely to perform spinal fusions than their neurosurgical colleagues. Some of those predisposed to using fusions liberally do so with far more ease than I think is appropriate, as you will see in a later chapter on spinal surgery. Recently, the distinction between neurosurgeons and orthopedists has blurred, as the new generation of spinal surgeons is trained in combined neurosurgical-orthopedic programs. However, orthopedic spine specialists are the only spine surgeons who treat complicated cases of scoliosis. Some orthopedists may use epidurals, and some now evaluate and treat low-back pain by performing discography and procedures to relieve discogenic pain. (I am always suspicious of the surgical skills of a spinal surgeon who doesn't devote himself mainly to truly invasive surgical procedures.)

Physiatrists specialize in the rehabilitation of the musculoskeletal and nervous systems and administer electrodiagnostic tests. They teach the use of exercise, prosthetic limbs, and body supports. They will also use physical therapy, including trigger-point injections. A small but growing number of physiatrists utilize interventional pain-management procedures, including nerve blocks, facet blocks, diskograms, and some radiofrequency lesioning procedures.

Primary-care physicians. Most PCPs are internists or family practitioners. If you have an acute pain from muscle spasm or other easily identifiable temporary pain, they can help you with conservative treatment and pain-relieving medications. Depending on your insurance, you may also need your PCP in order to get to a specialist.

Psychiatrists and psychologists naturally will use psychotherapy and behavioral techniques to help people cope with pain and its treatment. Psychiatrists may also prescribe medication to combat depression, anxiety, and, in some cases, the pain itself.

Radiologists do not evaluate pain problems but may be asked to perform facet blocks, nerve-root blocks, epidurals, and discograms. The problem with radiologists' performing these procedures is their lack of expertise in the diagnosis and treatment of painful disorders. Radiologists are usually not expert in deciding which patients should take medicine, which need rehabilitation, which need surgery, and which may benefit from diagnostic blocks or discography. I feel it is inappropriate for them to simply act as technicians, guided by the diagnostic concepts of their clinical colleagues. Would you want a surgeon to take out your appendix simply because your internist felt you had appendicitis and it needed to be removed? No. And you would not be likely to tolerate your neurologist's telling your neurosurgeon when and how to operate on your back. On the other hand, some interventional neuroradiologists inject material into the blood vessels that supply painful malignant tumors and blood-vessel malformations, procedures that can be very helpful in controlling pain. Only these specialized radiologists can safely perform these potentially dangerous procedures.

Rheumatologists treat arthritis, osteoporosis, and any disorders in bones, joints, or muscles, including diseases in which the body's immunity is turned against itself with crippling, painful consequences, as in rheumatoid arthritis. They prescribe medications, such as NSAIDs, muscle relaxants, narcotics, drugs to reduce an autoimmune response, and physical therapy. They also inject local anesthetics and steroids into painful joints in the extremities, temporarily reducing pain and inflammation.

Sports medicine specialists evaluate and treat sports injuries, including those of the spine. They are usually specialized physiatrists or orthopedic surgeons. When confronted with serious painful spinal disorders, they consult with spine specialists from the group above.

INTERVIEWING POTENTIAL DOCTORS

Once you've done the research and found doctors you believe might be able to help you, talk to them before you decide. Interview the doctor on the phone or in person. If you expect to have a lengthy conversation with the physician on the telephone, offer to pay for his or her time. I ask patients to fill out a detailed questionnaire (by mail or on my website) and send me their X-rays and other records to help me decide if I feel I can help them. Ask physicians question of this kind:

- How many patients with my physical complaint have you treated? (For common disorders, if they haven't treated hundreds, if not thousands, consider finding another doctor.)
- Were they treated with noninvasive, conservative methods, like medication, physical therapy, TENS, and acupuncture? Conservative measures should be tried for several weeks, barring a spinal emergency with excruciating pain that has not been well controlled by high doses of medication (including narcotics), severe or rapidly increasing weakness, and loss of sensation, or bowel and bladder dysfunction attributable to the spine.

- If that failed, what was the next step? If conservative methods fail, pain-relieving procedures may be considered for test-negative conditions, but surgery is usually required for pain and other neurological problems from ongoing pressure on spinal roots or the cord. (For patients with cancerous spinal tumors pressing on the roots or cord, radiation should be used instead of surgery in many cases.)

- How long should I undergo conservative treatment before trying invasive pain treatments, such as nerve blocks, radiofrequency lesioning, vertebroplasty (restoring bone by injecting liquid cement), implantable pumps, and invasive neurosurgical methods of pain control? (See the above answer. Invasive methods of pain control should usually not be used if your pain can be well controlled through well-tolerated medications, including chronically administered narcotics, taken orally or through skin patches. Lifestyle changes, including weight loss and alteration of exercise regimen and daily activities, should also be employed in relieving pain before trying procedures. Some people do not want to or cannot live on chronic medication; for them, pain-relieving procedures may be used. However, understand that even if a procedure to treat chronic pain was deemed successful by the standards of the profession and specialty, you may still require some pain medication afterward.

- What are the short- and long-term risks of treatment with medications or undergoing an invasive procedure? Make sure your doctor gives you a full review of all possible risks and balances them with benefits.

- Were most patients with conditions like mine
  significantly relieved or cured of their back pain?
  If not, what became of them?

Once your doctor has prescribed a treatment, ask about alternatives. If he or she resists answering your question, change doctors! You do have choices, though you may have to step outside your health-insurance system to get them.

Find out what the long-term results of this physician's treatment are and how they compare with results published by other doctors using the same methods in similar patients. Getting better for only a few hours, days, weeks, or even months from an invasive treatment that is designed to provide years of relief is not enough.

Talk with Other Patients

Ask your doctor for a list of references and ask for the names of patients for whom his or her treatments were successful and also for whom they were not. I provide these to my patients. If a doctor is offended by this idea, he or she may not be the right one for you. Ask these patients the following:

- Did the treatment really help?
- Was it worth the cost and inconvenience?
- How did the outcome change your life?
- What was the actual procedure like?
- What was the facility like where the procedure
  was performed?

By speaking to patients whose treatment failed, you will be able to tell how the physician manages such patients. Did the physician abandon them or direct them to another source of help?

You should have your own Plan B if your physician's proposed treatment plan proves ineffective. (However, remember that many chronic painful conditions cannot be cured, only significantly helped.) If you seem to be getting nowhere with one physician, consider finding another, if for nothing else than another opinion. Speaking to patients who had similar problems may guide you to another specialist. "May I speak to some who were not helped?" is a question you may want to ask at some point if your doctor's treatments appear to have no significant *long-term* effect. I have lost few patients to other colleagues in the medical system, except those I referred who moved out of the area, probably because my patients respect my opinion and my treatments are effective. However, I do have a list of people with whom I have been less successful than I desired, though not for lack of trying. I am on excellent terms with the vast majority of these patients—many are still in my practice—and can always request their help in talking with another patient.

WHAT YOU SHOULD KNOW ABOUT PAIN SPECIALISTS

The population of physicians practicing pain management exploded in the mid-1990s. There are well over four thousand of them in the United States, and they include a wide range of specialties. Pain specialists are advocates for those in chronic pain. They try to help their patients with medication, including narcotics; when appropriate, some perform or refer patients for pain-relieving procedures, such as radiofrequency lesioning, nerve blocks, laser, and other interventions you'll learn about in this book.

My one reservation is that as a group they too often feel

that pain management is an end in itself. As a result, they may fail to diagnose problems causing pain which surgery or other procedures can cure. Pain clinics thus often become the final resting ground of people who suffer from pain that other doctors cannot treat or relieve. Many physicians in these clinics simply try to use their tools to make you feel better rather than take a good second look to determine if your pain can be more definitely treated by, for example, surgery. If you have a hammer everything looks like a nail. If all a doctor does is give pain medication or perform blocks, that's all the patients will get.

I always tell my young medical residents to think outside the box in terms of both diagnosis and treatment. In real estate, location, location, location is key. In medicine, it's diagnosis, diagnosis, diagnosis. Much back pain is never relieved because its source is never fully diagnosed and therefore remains untreated. Whenever possible, a diagnosis must be made that may open the door to definitive treatment and liberation from the pain clinic. This is a path not always taken.

I want my residents to approach all patients with this in mind: "There are no intractable patients, only intractable physicians. Patients don't have intractable pain. You just don't know how to treat it."

Once a diagnosis is made, physicians and patients, in that order, must be realistic about what a treatment can and cannot achieve. Physicians are expected to educate their patients about what treatment is most likely to liberate them from the pain clinic. The primary goal of physicians treating pain should be the liberation of patients from pain clinics. This means less medication, fewer visits, and fewer procedures so you can eventually get to work and enjoy your life.

Key Points to Finding the Best Doctor

- If you have any doubts about a doctor's ability to treat your pain effectively, obtain a second opinion, even if you have to pay for it out of pocket.
- Be as accurate as you can in describing your pain and the treatment you have tried so far.
- Expect your doctor to take you seriously and believe that you are in pain.
- Be realistic in terms of outcome. Depending on your condition, you may have to live with some degree of chronic pain while taking medication.
- You do *not* have to live with moderately severe, much less excruciating, chronic pain.
- Most Americans who become disabled by pain don't have to. They received the wrong care or the right care too late.
- The goal of your physician should be to liberate you as much as possible from the medical system, a goal that is all too lacking in the treatment of chronic pain.

Chapter 5

How to Get and Pay
for the Best Treatment
for Back Pain

Most people with chronic back pain see several doctors before they find the one who can help them. Some, unfortunately, never find one. In today's health-care system you may not be covered for all the doctor visits and diagnostic tests you need in order to get to the bottom of the problem. Also, you may need treatment or medications that medical insurance does not cover. You have to learn to get around these road blocks.

It's crucial to understand what your health insurance covers. The diagnostic testing that may be best for you may be unavailable in your medical plan, especially in an HMO. Indeed, your doctor may fail to prescribe the best test or treatment because your insurance won't cover it. Or unnecessary tests or procedures may be prescribed in part because the insurance reimbursement is more lucrative. The doctors in your plan may not be the best to recognize and treat your condition.

Under the time constraints of managed care, doctors are so programmed that they have no time to notice the unusual.

One woman's painful disk was small and hard to detect on the poor-quality MRI from her health maintenance organization. This meant a doctor had to look carefully and take the time to add things up. The woman had recurrent back and right leg pain, identical to the symptoms of her previous disk herniation that were completely relieved when it was surgically treated. All of the physicians treating her should have examined carefully the area of the old disk herniation. If they had a problem interpreting the first, poor-quality MRI, they should have sent her to get a better one. But to have that expensive test redone, a physician would have to have taken the time to argue with the HMO administrative staff for the need for another scan. Many insurance companies will pay for diagnostic tests done only at a laboratory they choose, which may not be the best lab or one your doctor trusts.

Under this system, you often won't have the option of expensive tests that may pinpoint what is wrong with you and help you get the correct treatment quickly and aggressively before your problems escalate. If your doctor does want you to have tests, to call in a specialist, or to have a procedure, you and your doctor must be prepared to get precertification.

Consider trying to get a test or procedure precertified by your insurance carrier. This is a time-consuming administrative procedure that involves a detailed telephone interview with you and your doctor and the insurance company. It is a special request to allow payment for a procedure. This does not necessarily mean the company will pay for the test or procedure, but they will consider reimbursing you for it.

DO YOUR HOMEWORK

An HMO—health maintenance organization—is a plan that covers only approved doctors and medical facilities. A

PPO—preferred provider organization—allows you to go out of the network and be responsible for whatever the insurance company doesn't pay. Often out-of-network physicians do not accept insurance company copayment and are paid directly by the patient. Alternatively, the physicians may await the insurance company payment and then bill you for the balance. The premiums for HMOs are generally less than those for PPOs. (They are all expensive these days.) There are ways of finding better care even in an HMO. For example, if you live in an area with a highly respected hospital or medical center, find out if doctors in that center are included in your HMO. If it is a large center, it's possible that many of them are. Also, you have the option of finding other doctors within that medical center—and your plan—that may suit you better than others.

With your encouragement, I believe, most doctors, though unable to help you but willing to help you get an excellent second opinion, can guide you in the right direction. Remember that your physicians, like you, have grown accustomed to working within the system. If you're in trouble with chronic back pain, find a way to the most experienced physicians in the world, outside your insurance network if necessary.

How can you get the best possible care in the era of managed care? First, you must be willing to work to find and gain access to the best care, even if it is outside your network and town. Second, if you are not improving under a particular doctor's care or if the doctor recommends surgery, get a second opinion. You have choices to make. Should you pay an experienced physician outside your network to help you get long-lasting relief so that you can pick up and play with your children or grandchildren? It's your choice.

GETTING THE MOST FROM YOUR HEALTH-INSURANCE PLAN

Money does not always buy quality, but it helps. The least expensive doctors in your plan are not necessarily either the best or the worst. However, if you consult with an experienced specialist who charges enough money to be able to focus on your problems for sixty minutes, as opposed to one who sees two or three patients in that time, you are likely to receive better care.

If you have long-standing back pain that has not been adequately treated by physicians in your network or ones you consider affordable or geographically convenient, it may be time to look elsewhere and spend more money out of pocket. Patients covered by insurance plans that allow more choice rather than managed-care plans still have work to do. Many insurance companies balk at paying for high-quality tests to diagnose and treat many painful conditions, because many of them are test-negative (such as whiplash), and there are no objective tests to prove the severity of your pain.

Medications

Some insurers limit the amount of some pain-relieving drugs patients may obtain on their plan in a given period of time. Many insurance companies do not reimburse much for costly invasive pain-management procedures. For example, some policies will cover only two or three nerve blocks (diagnostic or therapeutic injections) in a year, even though you may need six to fully evaluate a painful spinal condition and another procedure, six radiofrequency lesions (destruction of nerves carrying pain signals), to obtain long-term pain relief. Current insurance policies often result in insufficient pain control, forcing you to spend your own money to get adequate pain relief.

Your doctor may help you appeal insurance company decisions, but ultimately it is you who has a contract with the insurance company and therefore must decide how to deal with the limitations of coverage. You may have to pay a small or even large portion of your doctor's fee out of your pocket to obtain the pain relief you desire. If you are self-employed, you may also choose to change plans.

Key Points about Paying for the Best Care

- Failing to obtain good care early in your illness may condemn you to a life of chronic physical and emotional pain, disability, reduced lifestyle, and financial hardships.
- If your health insurance company refuses to pay for particular tests or treatment that you need, make an appeal in writing.
- Consider changing your medical coverage to an insurer who gives you a choice of any medical care you want, even if it costs more.

Part II

Common Causes of Back Pain

Chapter 6

Muscle Injuries and Myofascial Back Pain

Muscle spasm is a common cause of acute back and neck pain. Many backs go into spasm following spring cleanup of the yard: overuse. Weekend warriors play sports without warming up first or conditioning their muscles. Result: They strain their backs. Others lift or pull heavy objects using their backs rather than their legs for leverage and cause a spasm. There are as many ways to hurt the muscles around the spine as there are people who put themselves out of action with this type of acute back pain. Muscles in any part of the spine can go into spasm, but the lower back is the most common area for spasm, as it is for disk herniations.

A muscle spasm is an involuntary local muscle contraction. It can be acute or chronic. It can be caused by repetitive overuse: raking and picking up autumn leaves. Or it can be caused by misuse and muscle injury, such as a sudden, poorly coordinated lunge to hit a tennis ball. It can also occur in response to an underlying painful problem, such as an acute disk herniation or chronic pain following failed spinal surgery.

Any awkward movement—misuse or injury—can lead to

a severe, painful muscle spasm and even cause the back to lock in place. Not only exertion; ordinary things like sneezing, coughing, bending to tie your shoe, or turning to face a different direction can cause a spasm. Finally, many of you who have had a disk herniation know how some of the muscles in the back or neck, occasionally in the leg or shoulder, go into painful spasm. Unlike the focal spasms of what is referred to as myofascial pain (described later in this chapter), this kind of spasm involves entire muscles, which is why your back can lock up with it.

Acutely damaged muscles become painful because acid and other toxic chemicals are produced within the muscle after overuse: a reaction to misuse or injury. Any spasm, regardless of the cause, can turn the muscles of the back into a hard, painful knot. You have likely had a severe back or neck spasm or know of someone who has; it literally keeps you from moving, as if you were in a painful, muscular cast.

Not only do injured muscles often go into spasm but chronically painful underlying spinal conditions, such as a disk herniation, can cause chronic spasm, worsening the underlying pain. Here the spasm is mediated by the nervous system; it is not due to muscle injury. Such a reflexive spasm is caused by excessive pain impulses traveling up the root compressed by the disk to the cord. Then, through a reflex mechanism there, other nerve impulses are sent back to the root, which results in spasm of the muscles supplied by it.

This reflex mechanism may be active even if the root is not compressed or irritated. For example, the pain from a broken vertebra or one damaged by a tumor may cause spasm of the muscles around it. In this case, both the vertebra and the affected muscles are supplied by the same roots. In these cases of reflex spasm, our muscles have formed a sort of splint to protect the underlying spine. Unfortunately, the splint may be as painful as the underlying problem.

Ongoing spasm, regardless of the cause, injures the muscle to some extent. However, once the underlying cause is removed, the spasm should diminish in at most a few days.

Straining Your Back

The difference between a strain and spasm may be academic when it comes to sore back muscles, since the treatment is similar. Strain is caused predominantly by overuse: repetitive, forceful movements that result in muscle soreness without spasm. Muscle is made up of individual and segmental strands of tissue. When any muscle, including those around the spine, encounter excessive pulling force, individual strands can stretch or tear—become strained—while the rest of the muscle remains intact. If you do lots of bending, lifting, and twisting, you are probably no stranger to this type of back pain. On the opposite side of the coin are people who rarely exercise. Muscles and ligaments become weak. When an inactive person suddenly becomes active, injuries are common.

The major symptom of back strain is pain when you stretch the muscle and you feel it tighten. If the strain is more severe, the symptoms are abrupt and immediately disabling. They are often accompanied by what patients describe as an audible snap or pop. After the initial burst of pain, symptoms of severe strains may subside, making them sometimes less painful than minor strains. Lumbar muscle strains may cause a broad, aching pain across the lower back or the pain may be limited to one side. You may have trouble bending down or standing up straight. You may also feel an occasional spasm when you move around or even while sleeping.

DIAGNOSING AND TREATING BACK MUSCLE INJURIES

First, do not try home treatment if in addition to pain, you have weakness, bowel or bladder problems, numbness, or tingling in your arms or legs. These suggest that you have more than a muscle problem and indeed suggest a disk herniation, broken vertebra, or spinal instability, resulting in the compression of the cord or nerve roots. For moderate-to-severe pain, see your doctor immediately. For what you interpret as just muscle pain, see your doctor if it persists for a month or so. Make sure your doctor gives you a thorough examination with appropriate high-quality tests, like an MRI, to see if there is damage to a spinal disk, a fracture, slippage, or an unsuspected cancer.

We can't see a spasm on X-ray or MRI, and it may not be detectable by many sophisticated diagnostic tests, but your doctor can diagnose it by touching the muscle in question and feeling the tightness.

A physical and neurological exam may include testing the range of motion by observing how you bend forward, backward, and from side to side. Nerve root irritation from a herniated disk may cause pain shooting down your leg when you raise it with your knee straight, as you lie on your back. This pulls the lower lumbar nerve roots against a disk fragment pressing on them, causing increased leg pain or sciatica.

Your doctor may recommend stronger pain medication, physical therapy, or, if your situation has a serious anatomical cause, surgical consultation.

Relax the Muscle

The goal of treatment for a spasm is to relax the muscle, reduce its need for food, bring blood to the area to flush out the irritating acid, and break the spasm-pain cycle. The best way to relieve spasms is to keep moving, but you should do this gradually. Increase your movements to see how far the muscle can stretch. Over several days to a few weeks, a combination of exercises and nonprescription medications—occasionally prescription drugs—will help relieve the spasm so the muscles will go back to their normal tension. However, spasm from an ongoing underlying painful cause, such as disk herniation or failed back surgery, is not likely to resolve unless the underlying source of pain heals or is successfully treated.

Ease the Pain with Medication

Tylenol is a good pain reliever to start with. You can also try nonsteroidal anti-inflammatory drugs (NSAIDs) like aspirin, ibuprofen (Advil), and naproxen (Aleve). If you have a history of reflux disease or ulcers, use the COX-2 inhibitors: Celebrex, Vioxx, or Bextra, for example. While they are no more effective than their older counterparts, they are less toxic on the gastrointestinal system. A muscle relaxant, such as Flexeril, Robaxin, and Valium, will calm spasm.

Use Heat and Stretching

While cold is useful in treating ankles and wrists, it usually is less effective than heat for spinal muscular pain. If you feel that cold is useful, put a cold pack of ice cubes wrapped in a towel on the sore spot soon after the pain begins. Do this several times a day for fifteen to twenty minutes.

Heat therapy will warm and relax sore tissues. You can get heat from a hot bath, a heating pad, liniment (such as Bengay or Tiger Balm), or by using hot wraps. Heat dilates the blood vessels of the muscles surrounding the spine, thus increasing the flow of oxygen and nutrients to the muscles, helping them to heal. Heat allows the muscles and soft tissue around the spine to stretch, reducing stiffness and increasing flexibility. (Heat is often used in physical therapy to prepare patients for gentle stretching exercises to increase flexibility.)

When combined with stretching, the benefits of heat therapy are greater than heat alone. Stretching exercises are appropriate self-care treatments to relieve the discomfort of back spasm and strain. Massage may also be temporarily beneficial because it increases blood flow to the painful muscle and loosens it.

Prevention

After you have strained a back muscle, it is more vulnerable to another injury. The only way you can change this fate is to change your lifestyle in a way that will avoid the causes. Exercise is important to strengthen your back and also your abdominal muscles, which help support your spine. Good posture while sitting, standing, and even sleeping helps, too. Learn how to lift and carry heavy items. Use ergonomics when sitting in chairs, wear a seat belt when traveling, and use protective equipment in sports. For more about preventing back pain, go to Chapter 21.

MYOFASCIAL PAIN

Low-back pain is a common symptom of myofascial pain syndrome (MPS). Myofascial or trigger-point pain *is perhaps the most common form of pain affecting the spine.* "Myo" refers to muscles and "fascia" is the tough coating, like Saran Wrap, that envelops our muscles. Many people have had this type of pain at one time or another without knowing its name. It is usually a reaction to lifestyle: overuse, such as from shoveling snow all day. Or it may also reflect a more serious underlying disease. It can be either acute or chronic.

The principal feature of myofascial pain is the trigger

point, a localized area of deep muscle tenderness accompanied by a palpable nodule in the muscle. Many cases of myofascial pain refer pain to a site distant from the trigger point.

Medical science has shown that structural problems, like tumors, disk herniations and damaged nerves, cause chronic pain. However, Dr. Janet Travell, known to the public as President Kennedy's physician, and her colleague, Dr. David G. Simons, expressed a theory that muscles themselves can cause pain from abnormalities, called trigger points, in bundles of muscle fibers. When poked, these small areas of muscle tenderness cause severe pain that often triggers a jump away from the poking finger. Thus, the name. The pain produced by this nasty, probing examining finger occurs both at the trigger point and in areas to which it is referred. Which area it will be can be defined with some certainty: for example, myofascial pain from the buttock produces both localized buttock soreness and referred pain down the leg that may mimic sciatica.

Myofascial pain may occur in a small muscle with few trigger points, such as one around the inner upper shoulder blade, or a large muscle, like that on the side of the thigh from the hip to the knee. The area of tenderness may range from a small knot of less than a square inch to a large area of many square inches. This is focal pain, as opposed to regional pain, which covers the whole back. Regional pain may also affect the back from the ribs down to the pelvis on both sides or one side of the neck from the head to the shoulder blades and the back of the shoulder.

Why You Get This Pain

Myofascial pain occurs equally in both sexes and affects all ages. It often accompanies muscle stiffness and fatigue and may plague you both while you are moving and at rest. However, this pain is different from the muscle spasm or strain mentioned above or the diffuse soreness of the flu. It appears to be caused by several factors, most commonly overuse or overstretching of unconditioned muscles. It is a form of pain common to workaholics who sit in a poor posture all day in front of a computer and couch potatoes who spend hours watching television while crippling their bodies. Weekend warriors abusing those sedentary bodies without sufficient warm-up are also prime candidates for myofascial pain.

Other medical problems can mimic or even cause myofascial pain, such as a torn muscle or some systemic diseases, including rheumatoid arthritis. Fibromyalgia can follow or coexist with myofascial pain. Even depression and anxiety can cause or exacerbate myofascial pain.

Underlying pain from the spinal disks and facet joints often causes myofascial pain in the muscles overlying the painful spinal structures. In people with one-sided lumbar-facet pain, myofascial pain of the buttock and upper thigh muscles is exceedingly common, as is bursitis of the covering of the hip joint. Unless all three sources of pain (facets, muscles, and bursa) are treated, they will not get better. Muscles supplied by nerves pinched by herniated disks can also develop myofasical pain on top of the pain from the pinched nerve.

Diagnosis Is Test-Negative

Myofascial pain is test-negative. There are no X-ray or electrical diagnostic tests that can confirm the diagnosis. Examining the trigger points under a microscope reveals no consistent abnormality, so diagnosis is purely clinical—based on your history and physical examination—especially finding trigger points in the muscle areas that are painful.

Unfortunately, many physicians consider this pain as not significant. For a few days, it may be annoying. If it lingers for several months and results in significant deterioration of your lifestyle and you feel you are stuck with a disbelieving doctor, find another who will find out why you have persistent pain.

Myofascial pain is a principal reason why people seek out chiropractic manipulation, which usually doesn't help, or massage and physical therapy, which do.

TREATING MYOFASCIAL PAIN

Noninvasive treatment includes hot wraps, drugs (nonsteroidal anti-inflammatory drugs, muscle relaxants, and antidepressants), TENS (transcutaneous electrical nerve stimulation), acupuncture, mild electrical stimulation of the overlying skin, and physical therapy. (See Chapters 16 and 20 for more on these techniques.) If necessary, these treatments may be used together. There are also three highly effective noninvasive or minimally invasive means of treating this condition, especially when used in concert with the above treatments.

Spray and stretch is an effective procedure of spraying a coolant over the skin overlying trigger points, followed by massaging or stretching the painful muscle. Since the spray-and-stretch procedure is less invasive than the trigger-point injections described below, some physicians prefer to try it first.

Trigger-point therapy is the injection of a local anesthetic, possibly mixed with a corticosteroid, into trigger points of tight muscles. It may relieve pain and return a sore muscle to normal functioning temporarily or permanently, depending on the cause of the pain and on the drugs used. Similar relief may be gained by dry-needling (inserting a needle into the trigger point) or injecting saline (sterile salt water, similar to body fluid). These procedures, however, may be more painful than the injection of local anesthetics. There have been no well-controlled studies of trigger-point therapy for back or limb pain. Nevertheless, it is widely used.

Botox injection is the new kid on the block. This technique is the injection of a minuscule amount of a nerve toxin. Used for medical purposes, this toxin causes a mild, focal-controlled muscle weakness (not paralysis) lasting three to four months and providing long-term relaxation of trigger points and relief from myofascial pain. Botox injections are an exciting therapy because of the long-lasting effect. However, Botox is expensive, and when used inappropriately, can cause excessive, though temporary, muscle weakness. It should not be used to treat myofascial pain unless nothing else works.

Success Is Up to You

Injections are not a substitute for physical therapy; they are an adjunct to it. Remember, the most important aspect of successful treatment for myofascial pain is you. The principal reason for correctly diagnosed myofascial pain to persist is the unwillingness or inability of the patient to do the stretching exercises required to treat it. They take weeks to months and are uncomfortable; you are stretching a painful, tight muscle. Moreover, patterns of myofascial pain are likely to recur in some people, perhaps because of the way they use their bodies in response to a slowly degenerating hip or a progressively arthritic neck. If your pain returns, get back to treatment and work at it.

The earlier you nip it in the bud, the easier it will be to relieve.

GLUTEUS MAXIMUS SYNDROME

This is an example of a myofascial pain problem that may result in buttock pain and perhaps mimic sciatica. The gluteus maximus is the powerful muscle of the buttock that helps you stand erect, walk, run, climb stairs, and rise from a seated position. It is attached to the coccyx at the base of your spine and the back of your pelvis. A spasm or tightness of this muscle can cause local buttock and even sciatica-like pain when you try to walk uphill in a bent-over position, pain on prolonged sitting, and in swimming the crawl. Normally, the spasm and pain are on only one side. Manual manipulation of the muscle often relieves this type of spasm, when combined with physical therapy and, if needed, trigger-point injections.

PIRIFORMIS SYNDROME

Deep inside the buttock is a muscle called the piriformis that originates on the sacral vertebrae and stretches to the thighbone. This muscle rotates your thigh outward when your upper leg is brought back behind you. The sciatic nerve runs under the piriformis muscle as it leaves the spinal canal and travels down the leg.

The piriformis can cause pain if it is overused, such as by repeatedly lifting things from the ground and throwing them over one shoulder—loading a truck with hay or firewood—or from running. Myofascial pain affecting the piriformis muscle will cause pain to radiate down the back of the thigh. Women may experience vaginal and pelvic pain during sexual intercourse. The pain is made worse when the muscle is stretched, as in bringing the leg, bent at the knee, across the center of the body.

Sometimes piriformis syndrome is associated with low-back pain or pain around the coccyx, groin, or over the hip. It is often associated with sacroiliac-joint-related pain (see Chapter 15), which must be recognized and treated apart from the piriformis syndrome. One-sided facet pain may also coexist with either piriformis syndrome or sacroiliac-joint pain, as may bursitis of the hip. They all have to be recognized and treated separately, and they can be, with good, lasting results.

Diagnosis and Treatment

Piriformis syndrome is diagnosed from the history and physical examination. Whether the symptoms are from myofascial pain or entrapment (see next section), they cannot in the office be completely differentiated from lower lumbar nerve pain from disk herniation or stenosis. Spinal-root compression must be excluded before the diagnosis of piriformis syndrome can become a prime target of treatment (root compression can coexist with myofascial pain of various muscles). Obviously, a disk herniation, which may be the underlying cause of myofascial pain and require surgery as the best treatment, should be recognized and dealt with before embarking on a host of trigger-point injections and physical therapeutic measures for focal muscle spasm.

Treatment of this disorder is the same as for any myofascial pain—stretching exercises, analgesics, anti-inflammatory medications, and muscle relaxants. For persistent pain, trigger-point injections of local anesthetics and corticosteroids in the muscles followed by stretching exercises may be used with good result.

SCIATIC-NERVE ENTRAPMENT

A separate issue from the problem of myofascial pain is sciatic-nerve entrapment by the piriformis. Some contend that in some patients the piriformis muscle and underlying sciatic and some other nerves and blood vessels are so positioned that the muscle irritates or compresses these nerves, causing sciatic, groin, and hip pain. People with this problem will have symptoms of sciatic-nerve irritation, including tingling, which is at times painful, involving the affected sciatic nerve, not just pain in the buttock or thigh (they may have that, too). This diagnosis accounts for at most a small percentage of patients with buttock, hip, and sciatic pain usually from other causes. I am unimpressed by the outcomes of its usual treatment: surgical decompression of the sciatic nerve under the muscle. The vast majority of patients treated surgically for this purported diagnosis still have chronic pain postoperatively, probably because the entrapment was never the true cause of it.

Diagnosis

In entrapment, electrodiagnostic tests may document nerve compression in the area of the buttock, and an MRI scan may detect an enlarged muscle inside the pelvis. However, I remain unconvinced that this entity is the real culprit in most patients with this diagnosis. The recommended treatment for what may be considered piriformis entrapment is surgical decompression of the affected nerves and nearby blood vessels. In general, I advise against this therapy.

Key Points to Treating Muscle Spasm and Myofascial Pain

- Never ignore muscle pain accompanied by weakness, numbness, and bowel or bladder problems.
- We cannot see a muscle spasm or sprain on X-ray or MRI. Your doctor can diagnose either by touching the muscle and feeling the tightness.

- Heat dilates the blood vessels to increase the flow of oxygen to muscles, helping them heal.
- After you have strained a back muscle, that muscle is more vulnerable to another such injury.
- Low-back pain is a common symptom of myofascial pain syndrome.
- Trigger points—areas of deep muscle tenderness accompanied by a palpable nodule in the muscle— are the principal feature of myofascial pain syndrome.
- Other medical problems can mimic or cause myofascial pain. They include small muscle tears, systemic rheumatological diseases, and fibro-myalgia.
- Pain from spinal disks and facets often causes spasm and myofascial pain in the muscles overlying those structures.
- The principal reason that myofascial pain persists is the unwillingness of the patient to do the stretching exercises required to treat it.

Chapter 7

Facet Syndrome: Painful Spinal Joints

Many people are unaware that they have joints in their spines. There are two tiny facets one on each side of each vertebra to keep the spine stable. As do the shoulder and the knee, spinal facets join two bones: the vertebra above and below. Spinal facets are true synovial joints. They have a capsule (synovium) that is lubricated by fluid and are filled by a network of pain-sensitive nerve fibers. These small, delicate joints are prone to injury, deterioration, and, in some diseases, inflammation, and they sometimes become sources of chronic neck and back pain independent of the disks and spinal nerves. After muscle pain, facet pain is probably the most common cause of low-back pain.

Lumbar-facet pain is the most common (though facet pain can occur in any part of the back). The telling sign of lumbar-facet pain is back and possibly buttock, groin, and thigh pain, especially while sitting or arching your back, which increases the pressure on the facets in the back of the spine. Bending forward or lying down usually relieves lumbar-facet pain.

Cervical-facet pain is the second most common facet problem and may cause headaches, shoulder, and occasionally arm pain. These facets are often more painful when the neck is bent backward or to the sides, which increases pressure on the facets. Headache from facet pain (cervicogenic headache) occurs in the morning after a night of tossing and turning, which also increases pressure on these joints.

Thoracic-facet pain is less common. These joints become injured when excessive amounts of rotation and extension cause a sharp pain anywhere between the upper shoulder blade and the area over the lower ribs. Pain from thoracic facets doesn't usually travel to the side or front of the chest. Thoracic vertebrae form a relatively immobile segment of the spine compared to the highly mobile neck and lumbar area. Therefore, the thoracic disks and facets are less likely to wear out. As you will see below, disk degeneration helps cause facet pain.

How Facet Pain Develops

The vertebral bodies, separated by the disks, make up the front of the spine and carry the weight of the structure. As the disks degenerate, the facets end up carrying more weight than they should, leading them to wear down and become painful. When facets wear out they can become arthritic, just as occurs in other joints, such as the knees, hips, or fingers.

Osteoarthritis usually develops in the facets of the neck and lower back. The synovium wears out, bone surfaces rub together, and the facets become painful. With time, calcified outgrowths, called osteophytes, develop around the facets, degenerated disks, and supporting ligaments of the spine. The result is loss of flexibility and possibly pain.

Being overweight is an increasingly common cause of problems with lumbar facets. Heavy people wear down their disks earlier and therefore may develop chronic facet pain—

among other spinal problems—early in their lives. This is reflected in the well-known Framingham Study, which has followed the health of female residents of a Massachusetts town for more than fifty years. Young women who are overweight were more likely than their thinner neighbors to develop arthritis later in life. The heaviest women were twice as likely to get it as slimmer ones.

Facets can be injured from trauma, such as whiplash from a rear-end auto collision (see the next chapter). They can also be injured in sports, such as by being tackled in football or falling off a horse. Golfers are prime candidates for lumbar and thoracic facet injury because of the repetitive twisting motions as they swing the club. A sudden excessive movement—especially backward or to the side—can traumatize the joint and cause pain that can last several days. Sometimes this pain becomes chronic, for reasons that are poorly understood.

Spondylolisthesis or slippage of one vertebra over another can also cause low back pain from the facets and other structures. Pain can be controlled by treating the facets only if the slippage is of a low degree (a few millimeters at most) and the spine is relatively stable. If the vertebrae wiggle significantly, facet treatment won't be enough. Medication and lifestyle modification may help you to tolerate your back pain; if they don't, surgery—fusion—is needed to stabilize your spine.

The Thorny Problem of One-Sided Facet Pain

Often facet pain occurs on only one side of the spine. This is most common and troublesome in the lumbar spine and is difficult to treat. Part of the impediment to successful treatment is the multifaceted nature of this pain. This so-called one-sided lumbar-facet pain is often accompanied by pain in structures other than the facets. These pain generators may not be recognized and treated.

For example, one-sided lumbar-facet pain is often accompanied by myofascial pain in the buttock muscles and those overlying the hip on the side of the painful back. The sacroiliac joint on that side may be painful, as may be the trochanteric bursa, a fluid-filled sac overlying the hip joint, reducing friction from the muscles sliding over the joint. Distinct from the painful facets, these may be painful when you lie on them in bed. So the facets cause pain during the daytime and the other structures disturb sleep at night.

A second obstacle in treating one-sided lumbar pain successfully is recognizing and eliminating the often subtle, long-standing imbalances in posture and gait that created the problem. They may be deeply ingrained. One-sided lumbar pain may also be the result of less subtle gait disturbances, such as limping from an ankle, knee, or hip injury. Sometimes people with one-sided low-back pain walk or hold themselves in a slightly lopsided way, perhaps from habitually carrying a heavy briefcase or purse on that side. This is more correctable than the other orthopedically based reasons above.

These imbalances of stance and gait, whether subtle or evident, may cause lumbar and, occasionally, musculoskeletal structures higher up in the body, on one or both sides, to become excessively worn or painful. One-sided lumbar pain is worse when bending backward or to the affected side.

One-sided cervical-facet pain may arise after a fall or whiplash injury. It is less complicated to recognize and treat than one-sided lumbar pain. Less recognized by many doctors is one-sided thoracic-facet pain. This may arise for no discernible reason, or it may develop after a fall or from developing scoliosis. It is amenable to treatment if diagnosed and is usually less complicated than the one-sided lumbar-facet problem.

DIAGNOSING FACET PAIN

Facet problems are identified by the pattern of referred pain, local tenderness over the site, and pain in certain body positions. Your doctor will try to find the pain by poking or moving the suspected painful areas during a physical exam. (The complicated problem of one-sided pain is discussed above.) Physical examination should reveal tenderness over the affected facets and possibly painful trigger points in overlying or nearby muscles and in one-sided lumbar pain, possibly pain in the sacroiliac joint and bursa overlying the hip on the same side as the painful facets.

To make the diagnosis of facet pain and accompanying myofascial or other test-negative pain and to exclude other possible anatomically based causes of pain, it may be necessary to have a CT or MRI of the painful areas of the spine and, possibly, of the painful pelvis and hip.

Chronic facet pain may come from long-term changes in the joint, detectable by radiological studies, even though facet pain itself is not. *Normal appearing facets may hurt, and those that appear arthritic may not.* Therefore, facet pain is a test-negative condition, one whose diagnosis is made clinically (using the history and examination), not by radiological or other conventional studies. Many physicians incorrectly believe a joint that appears to be normal on studies such as CT scans or MRIs cannot be painful. Moreover, many neurologists and some neurosurgeons don't even consider painful facets as a cause of back pain. If they can't see something causing pressure on a nerve root or an unstable spine, they usually cannot diagnose the cause of pain.

The diagnosis of facet pain must be confirmed by the

patient's response to a diagnostic injection: a block of the facet or the nerves supplying it. This is not considered a routine test.

TREATING FACET PAIN

An acute episode of facet pain can be treated with rest, acetaminophen (Tylenol), NSAIDs, possibly stronger analgesics in the narcotic family, muscle relaxants if the muscles overlying the facets are in spasm, and, later, postural correction by a physical therapist. Heat treatment and massage to relax any muscle spasm may also be helpful. The mentholatum arthritis patch is a hydrogel formation that contains methyl salicylate, which provides deep penetrating heat to relieve sore joints and muscles. It may help some spine-related pain and overlying muscle spasm.

You may need injections of local anesthetics and corticosteroids into any especially painful muscles with trigger points (myofascial pain) associated with the facet problem. If relevant, the bursa overlying the hip may also be injected before starting to exercise. This needed exercise may be painful for the first few weeks. Additional therapies usually won't be needed.

Treatment of Chronic Facet Pain with Injections

Diagnosis and preliminary treatment of chronic facet-related pain can be done by injections into the facets or the nerves supplying these joints. Just as epidural injections are used to treat root pain within the spinal column (see Chapter 18), facet-joint injections are sometimes used to diagnose and, for the short term, treat pain from the facet joints. If the facets are in fact the sole or a major cause of pain, injections of anti-inflammatory corticosteroids and local anesthetics directly into the joints or over the nerves transmitting pain impulses from the facets to the spinal cord may reduce pain and facilitate rehabilitative therapy.

Injections are done under fluoroscopic or CT-scan guidance, sometimes after intravenous sedation, so that the needle can be placed exactly in the joint or over the nerve to the joint. The injection of anesthetic briefly blocks the pain signals emanating from the joint, and the corticosteroid reduces any inflammation of the joint and surrounding structures. The local anesthetic effect is used to confirm the diagnosis—based on your history and examination—of facet-related pain. This block lasts forty-five minutes to several hours, depending on the anesthetic used. The corticosteroid effect may last from several days to a few weeks.

Radiofrequency Therapy

A more lasting treatment to relieve pain from facet syndrome is radiofrequency therapy. This minimally invasive outpatient surgical technique destroys the nerves that supply the facet joint by a precisely delivered, localized application of heat. Radiofrequency lesioning should relieve facet-related pain for over two years. If the pain recurs, the treatment can be repeated. However, it cannot get rid of the cause of the pain: facet-joint degeneration. The correctly performed procedure can itself increase back pain for several weeks, but I have never met a working patient who could not go to work the day following these lesions, sometimes with the help of some pain relievers.

In some patients, lesions may result in patchy numbness—for less than three months—or mild supersensitivity of the skin of the back that is affected by the lesioned nerves.

Even when the procedure is done properly, not all the sources of pain may be reached. Fifty percent reduction of pain on a long-term basis is considered a good outcome.

Patients often ask me if they can hurt themselves by overdoing physical activities after a successful radiofrequency treatment. No. If they overdo it and herniate a disk or fall and break a facet, they will still experience severe pain. But in practical terms, they cannot hurt their arthritic facet joints by living a more active physical existence. For more about how this treatment is done, see Chapter 18.

Treating One-sided Facet Pain

Failure to recognize the accompanying pain-generators of one-sided lumbar-facet pain will result in a partially treated problem, producing chronic pain. If the facet is made less painful but the myofascial pain in the buttock, hip bursitis, or painful sacroiliac joint are left untreated, the patient will continue to experience pain. They won't care that their physician informs them that the pain no longer is coming from the facets.

In one-sided pain from asymmetrical weight-bearing, switching the side on which weight is carried or using a briefcase on wheels and engaging in exercise and physical therapy that builds up muscles on both sides of the lumbar area, buttocks, and hips can restore you to a comfortable existence.

For those with the more difficult to treat one-sided facet pain, after a good pain-relieving response to appropriate diagnostic blocks of the nerves that affect the facets, I lesion these nerves. If the sacroiliac joint appears to be painful, I initially block it or some of the nerves from the lower sacrum. If these blocks produce a good response, I lesion some of the nerves to part of the joint, usually with good results. I send patients with myofascial pain and bursitis for physical therapy before I inject them with local anesthetic and corticosteroids so they understand what to work on after the injections. Then I inject trigger points in the muscles of the buttock that allow the hip and leg to rotate outward; they are often affected by myofascial pain in one-sided lumbar-facet pain. Then if the bursa overlying the hip is tender, I also inject it. Following the injections, I send my patients back to physical therapy or, if they are highly motivated and understand the reason for the exercises, home, so they can exercise by themselves.

In patients with a significantly poor gait, the pain is more difficult to treat. A woman who had pain in her right lower back and buttock had difficulty walking for about two years, following a bad fracture of her right ankle. The ankle eventually required fusion, so it could no longer bend. This resulted in a severe permanent limp. That in turn brought on a right-sided facet syndrome with the other attendant problems so often accompanying this condition. Like many patients with one-sided facet pain, she responded to treatment but not as well as someone with facet pain emanating from both sides. She waddled like a duck when she walked, placing a tremendous strain on the right lumbar spine, buttock muscles, sacroiliac joint, trochanteric bursa, hip and knee joints, all of which hurt her. I could only do so much to keep her comfortable with her totally unnatural human gait. Eventually, her waddling created pain on the left side as well, a less severe mirror image of the right side.

Key Points about Facet Pain

- Facets are small joints, one on each side in the back of the spine, that connect two vertebrae.
- Facets keep your spine stable but are not made to bear considerable weight.
- Facets forced to bear weight as the disks degenerate are prone to deterioration.

- After muscle spasm, facet pain is probably the most common cause of low-back pain.
- Facet pain can occur anywhere in the spine. It is most common in the lower back.
- Facets that appear normal on radiologic studies may hurt, while those that appear arthritic may not.
- Osteoarthritis can develop in the facets of the neck and lower back.
- Being overweight causes problems with lumbar facets sooner rather than later.
- Radiofrequency lesioning of the nerves to the facets may relieve pain for two or more years.

Chapter 8

Chronic Whiplash Pain

After more than two decades of debate, whiplash is still a highly charged, emotional issue and continues to be the most controversial medical condition. Whiplash is the rapid bending forward and extension backward of the spine, usually the cervical spine, by an abrupt change in the speed and direction in which you are traveling in a moving vehicle. The most common cause of whiplash is being in a car that is rear-ended. The vehicle that hits the car you are in is obviously traveling faster than yours. When the collision occurs, your car is projected forward, forcing your head backward. Then your car rapidly decelerates, hits another car ahead of you, or you slam on the brakes to avoid it, and your head is thrown forward. All this may occur within seconds and cause damage to the facets and their coverings, disks, and the muscles around and the ligaments supporting the spine.

The whiplash may also cause the brain to bounce back and forth inside the skull. The brain is a mass of nerve and other cells and blood vessels. It has the consistency of moderately firm butter and is supported by leatherlike sheets (dura) and surrounded by a leatherlike sac filled with spinal fluid. At the base of the brain, delicate nerves, a fraction of an inch in diameter, leave the buttery mass, enter holes in the skull, then travel to your nose, eyes, ears, and other structures. You can readily understand that as a result of severe whiplash, in which the brain is thrown back and forth inside the dural sac inside the skull, damage to it and the nerves leaving it may occur. A whiplash injury may cause a mild concussion, which can affect thinking and mood. It can result in loss of hearing or balance and sense of smell. Double vision, ringing in the ears, and headaches are common. If the speed at which this accident occurs is high enough, broken vertebrae, a damaged spinal cord, and severe concussion or even a contusion or bruise of the brain, resulting in bleeding within it, can result. There are usually no broken bones, disk herniations, large blood clots, ripped muscle, or torn skin. The result of a whiplash injury is obviously painful, and the painful aftereffects, for unclear reasons, last varying times in different people.

Chronic Facet Pain

According to the National Institute of Arthritis and Musculoskeletal and Skin Diseases (NIAMS), more than 1.8 million people in the United States suffer from chronic pain and disability from motor vehicle accidents each year. The majority of these begin with minor neck injury. While most of the people heal in a matter of weeks, 20 percent to 40 percent have symptoms that are sometimes debilitating and persist for years. In one study of people with chronic pain from whiplash, most developed pain within three days of the accident and suffered from it for an average of more than four years. Of this group, 58 percent were women and 42 percent men. More than half had painful facets.

Acute whiplash pain may cause local or widespread muscle spasm. For those with chronic pain, the facets are the usual culprits, although muscle spasm may still exist. The top three segments of facets, C_{2-3}, C_{3-4}, and C_{4-5}, are responsible for head and upper neck pain. Lower facets may cause mid-to-lower neck, thoracic, and lumbar pain, as explained in the previous chapter.

Whiplash injury may also cause what we call discogenic pain. Even when not herniated, disks may have a torn covering (annulus) and internal tears within the nucleus. The torn annulus can be seen on MRIs. Not all disks with a torn annulus are painful (see Chapter 10). The C_{2-3} and C_{3-4} disks may cause headache and these and the C_{4-5} disks may also cause upper neck pain. Like facets, lower disks may cause lower neck, thoracic, or lumbar pain. Discogenic and facet pain may coexist.

SYMPTOMS OF WHIPLASH

Symptoms may occur right after the injury or may be delayed for several days. They include:

- neck pain and stiffness
- headaches
- pain in the shoulder or between the shoulder blades
- pain, numbness, or tingling (paresthesia) in the arm and/or hand
- less commonly, low-back pain, with possible radiation into the buttocks, groin, hips, and thighs

Symptoms of concussion, often caused by whiplash, include:

- dizziness
- ringing in the ears or blurred vision

- difficulty concentrating or remembering
- irritability
- sleep disturbance
- fatigue
- loss of libido
- depression

THE DIFFICULTY OF DIAGNOSING WHIPLASH

Whiplash often results in classic test-negative chronic pain so has become a big problem for both patients and insurers. Diagnosis is usually impossible to substantiate even with sophisticated radiological studies, such as high-quality MRI or electrophysiological tests, because the effects of whiplash on the body often cannot be traced.

Because soft tissue—muscle and ligament—injuries elsewhere in the body heal completely within a few months, it is often assumed that symptoms that persist even after a physical examination shows the patient to be normal and negative radiological studies must be caused by outside factors. The late whiplash syndrome has become one of the most controversial conditions in medicine. Some attribute the persistent symptoms to unresolved injury, while others blame them on underlying psychological factors or the possibility of financial gain. The insurance business constantly tries to prove that people with whiplash are malingerers, interested only in receiving compensation.

For patients suffering from chronic pain following whiplash, their problem is not only real but potentially disabling. Effective treatment for most of the causes of this kind of pain is available, provided the causes are diagnosed. Such causes are often inadequately diagnosed or treated, with possibly devastating results for the patient and those close to them.

I can tell you from personal experience with many patients

just how real this condition—and the pain—is. I testified in a trial in which a big automobile manufacturer had to pay a million and a half dollars to a man who was so damaged by whiplash—the car's headrest broke in an accident—that he developed chronic severe neck and head pain, permanent ringing in the ears, dizziness, balance difficulties, complete loss of the sense of smell, loss of libido, and an inability to function cognitively at the same level as he did before the accident; he could no longer work as a high-level accountant. His earning power was severely curtailed, he was in chronic pain, his social life was a ghost of what it had been, and despite psychiatric medication, he was understandably depressed.

Why We Can't Prove It

How whiplash occurs is well understood, but the extent and type of injuries vary. When we diagnose whiplash, other physically serious injuries, such as broken bones or damage to the nervous system, must be ruled out by a detailed neurological examination, CT scans and MRIs, and, possibly, electrophysiological tests.

We can't prove that someone has neck pain and headaches from whiplash because we can't see the damage that is causing the pain. However, how do you prove someone has a headache? In the vast majority of cases you can't. Most people with headaches don't have large brain tumors or hemorrhages that can be verified with an MRI or CT scan. Headaches and neck pain from whiplash must be accepted as a possible result of such an injury, diagnosed, and effectively treated.

The typical whiplash-related headache is often completely or in part referred pain from painful but not fractured or visibly torn cervical structures. This type of headache is called a cervicogenic headache. It typically involves pain radiating from the base of the skull in the back of the head up to the front of the head over the eyebrows or over the side of the head above the ears. It may exist on either or both sides. Often, the headache and accompanying neck pain may come on during sleep or are noted on awakening. This is due to the wear and tear on the neck structures by tossing and turning during sleep that may increase neck pain and stimulate cervicogenic headache. This neck and head pain may continue throughout the day, depending on a patient's tendency to experience headaches, severity of the problem, and lifestyle. For example, making much use of the side mirrors while driving to work may exacerbate such headaches.

TREATING ACUTE CERVICAL WHIPLASH PAIN

Since most whiplash injuries affect the neck, the balance of this chapter will focus on that structure, as opposed to the lumbar spine, which is affected less often. The lumbar spine can be treated in much the same manner as the neck, if appropriate, with good results.

Most whiplash-caused head and neck pain goes away in a few weeks to a few months. In the past, whiplash was often treated by immobilizing the neck in a cervical collar; today, we encourage early movement rather than keeping the neck rigid. The collar is best used intermittently for short periods.

In the first twenty-four hours after injury, apply heat and keep moving the neck slowly and gently. Your doctor may give you a series of exercises you can do at home. Return to work and normal activity as soon as you can bear to do so. No single treatment has proven effective, but exercises, physical therapy, chiropractic manipulation, cervical collars, massage, acupuncture, TENS, traction, ultrasound heat, ice, medication, and various kinds of injections have all helped some people some of the time.

Over-the-counter analgesics, such as acetaminophen (Tylenol), may be tried, as may mild-to-moderate-strength nonnarcotic prescription medication, such as NSAIDs (non-steroidal anti-inflammatory drugs), muscle relaxants, and tramadol (Ultram) or tramadol combined with acetamino-phen (Ultracet). Finally, narcotic analgesics may have to be used for several weeks to months. This category includes acet-aminophen and codeine (Tylenol No. 3), hydrocodone and acetaminophen (Vicodin or its relatives), oxycodone and acetaminophen (Percocet), other short-duration narcotics (morphine) and even long-duration narcotics (Oxycontin, MS Contin, Kadian, Duragesic). Chapter 17 has more details on these drugs.

Your doctor may prescribe isometric exercises as your condition improves. Symptoms disappear within a few months for about 75 percent of people who had whiplash. The other 25 percent need more complex medical treatment.

TREATING CHRONIC PAIN OR LATE WHIPLASH SYNDROME

The treatment of chronic neck pain after a whiplash injury (late whiplash syndrome) is difficult and often frus-trating to both patient and physician. Some patients with a whiplash injury never completely recover. There are many claims for various therapies for significant chronic pain from whiplash injury but little proof of their success. People have used the above treatments for acute pain. However, as the pain continues to linger, the doctor turns to more inva-sive treatments: facet injections, epidural injections, nerve blocks of various kinds, even surgery. The Quebec Task Force Study on Whiplash-Associated Disorders (WAD) was begun in 1989 to determine the clinical, public health, social, and financial determinants of WAD. As reported in the *New England Journal of Medicine* in 1996, the study found almost no literature to justify the use of facet injections for the treatment of whiplash. Surgery is also unlikely to do anything for whiplash-caused neck pain, and it may cause postoperative pain and permanently change your anatomy. Your objective in seeking treatment for any chronically painful disorder should be to liberate yourself as much as possible from the medical system, including the pain clinic.

In well over half of patients with chronic neck pain of this type, the pain originates in the cervical-facet joints. Myofascial and discogenic pain of long standing also contribute to chronic pain following whiplash. However, myofascial pain—focal spasm in a large area of muscle tightness—is often a reflection of underlying facet or discogenic pain. Therefore, simply treating the tight muscles with physical therapy, trigger-point injections, and muscle relaxants may fail to bring long-term relief. If pain originates below the muscles, it must be diagnosed. Although these deep pain-generators cannot be diagnosed radiographically, they can be identified by blocks directed against the nerves supplying the facets or by discography. Facet blocks may not be beneficial in the long term as therapy for facet-related pain, but diagnostic facet blocks or a block of the nerves supplying them, which is safer than blocks of the joints and equally effective, is a good means of confirming a clinical suspicion that the facets are generators of chronic pain.

The treatment for chronic facet pain is radiofrequency lesioning of the nerves to the painful facets. In my practice, this procedure applied to patients with cervical-facet pain from whiplash injury gives over two years of relief to over 80 percent of patients. (See the previous chapter.)

If discography demonstrates that one or several disks contribute to the pain, I have found that a series of radiofrequency lesions, done in one procedure within the disk itself, can give excellent relief, similar in degree and duration to lesioning the nerves to the facets. This is the only technique for dealing with cervical discogenic pain. Other techniques—IDET and laser treatment—to treat discogenic pain may be applied only to the large disks of the lumbar spine; these techniques use probes too large to be inserted into the small cervical disks.

Key Points about Whiplash

- Whiplash is one of the most controversial conditions in medicine.
- It is most frequently caused by a rear-end auto accident.
- Most whiplash heals in a matter of weeks, but 20 percent to 40 percent persist for years.
- It can lead to chronic neck, back, and head pain.
- Cervical facets and muscle spasm cause the pain.
- Whiplash can also cause discogenic pain.
- Because it is test-negative, others frequently don't believe that you have it.
- Diagnosis must be done by ruling out all other possibilities.
- It is treated with medication and radiofrequency lesioning.

Chapter 9

Pain from Spinal-Disk Herniation

As we age and our spinal disks begin to dry out, shrink, and become less stable, they can herniate, lose their covering, press on a nerve, and cause all manner of trouble. A herniated disk is an extrusion of a piece of the nucleus (the gel-like center) through a tear in the annulus (the tough, leatherlike outer cover). Most disk ruptures occur between ages thirty and forty; the disks still contain a normal amount of gel, but the annulus is beginning to wear out. If the gel remains inside the cover, it is a disk protrusion. If it escapes through a torn annulus, it is a disk extrusion. Extruded pieces of disk may move up or down the spinal canal a quarter to a half-inch or so from the area of herniation. Disks may protrude to the front, the sides, or to the back.

Most disk herniations occur in areas where the spine is maximally bent forward. The forward bending of these segments results in the vertebral bodies coming closer together toward the spinal canal than in the front of the spine. This places more stress on that part of the annulus and disk facing the spinal canal. The lower neck and the lowermost lumbar spine cause the most problems. Lumbar disks are herniated several times more frequently than their cervical counterparts. Presumably, this is because of greater weight on the lumbar spine. Thoracic herniations are rare; those causing problems are even less frequent. Disk herniations may be preceded by a history of intermittent episodes of back or neck pain, possibly with twinges in the leg or arm. This is from the annulus's being stretched and under tension. After the disk fully herniates, the pain increases and is usually accompanied by pain radiating down the leg or arm, depending on which root or roots are irritated.

The late actor Gregory Peck told a story about his back in his last magazine interview. As a young actor in New York he was in a body-movement class with the choreographer Martha Graham. He was sitting on the floor with his legs spread out trying to touch his feet with his head. Graham, a tough taskmaster, came up behind him and said, "Come on, Greg, you can do better than that." She pushed his back down and "put my back out." Peck said he wore a canvas brace for several years after that. What Peck may have had was a herniated disk. Let's hope you won't have the same experience.

If a herniated disk does compress a nerve root, it can cause not only pain but also possible weakness, numbness, and loss of normal reflexes in the area supplied by the root. Cervical- or thoracic-herniated disks can compress the spinal cord, and the large lumbar disks can significantly compress the cauda equina. (See figures 5 and 6.) These herniations can result in arm (cervical disks) or leg (lumbar disks) weakness, numbness below the area of the cord or cauda equina compressed by the disk, and bowel and bladder disturbance. Significant compression of the cauda equina usually also causes severe pain in

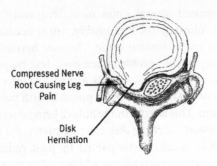

Compressed Nerve
Root Causing Leg
Pain

Disk
Herniation

FIGURE 5. Top view of lumbar spine.

both legs. Depending on the extent of deficit caused by this type of herniation, emergency neurosurgical decompression may be required to minimize the damage to the nervous system and prevent the creation of permanent nerve damage.

Disk herniations are common; 70 percent to 80 percent improve with time and care. Some herniate and heal, then herniate and heal again. Too often, however, people rush to have unnecessary surgery. They then may spend the rest of their lives repairing the repair.

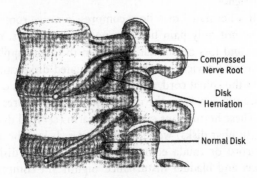

Compressed
Nerve Root

Disk
Herniation

Normal Disk

FIGURE 6. Side view of lumbar spine.

Cervical Disks

Cervical-disk herniations are less common than lumbar-disk herniations even though you move your neck more often than you do your lower back. There is substantially less weight in the neck than in the lumbar area. Nevertheless, because the cervical spine has a smaller internal diameter—canal—and smaller foramen than other parts of the spine, small herniations are more likely to impinge on a spinal root and cause pain to radiate down the arm. Numbing and tingling may occur as far down as the fingertips. The pain is usually most severe when the disk first herniates and compresses the root (or roots, depending on the anatomy). A cervical-disk herniation into the canal can also damage the spinal cord.

- Herniation of the C_{4-5} disk can affect the C_5 nerve root. This causes pain in the neck and over to the side of the shoulder and weakness in the other shoulder muscles and in the muscle that bends the elbow. The biceps reflex may be reduced. Sensory changes, such as numbness and tingling, may also occur in the deltoid area, on the side of the shoulder.
- Herniation of the C_{5-6} disk affects the C_6 root. This can cause pain running from the neck down the arm and hand to the thumb and forefinger. Weakness of some shoulder muscles, the biceps, and the wrist muscles that bend the wrists down and to the inside may exist. Sensory changes, along with pain, may extend to the lower arm and the thumb side of the hand. The biceps reflex may be reduced. This is one of the most common results of a cervical-disk herniation.

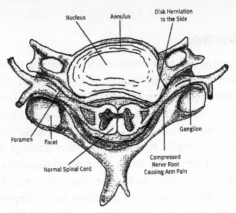

FIGURE 7. Disk herniation: Top view of cervical spine.

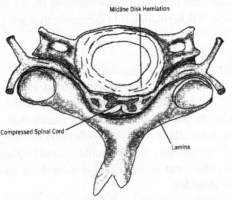

FIGURE 8. Disk herniation: Top view of cervical spine.

- Herniation of the C_{6-7} disk affects the C_7 root. Like the previous level, this is also a common site of disk herniation. Pain may radiate down to deep in the forearm and into the middle finger, and sensory changes may occur in the same area. Damage to this root causes weakness in the muscle that bends the wrist down and inward, other muscles that bend the wrist downward, and those that bend the finger, the triceps, and the muscles that raise the wrist inward, and some muscles that straighten the fingers. The triceps reflex may be reduced.

- Herniation of the C_7-T_1 disk affects the C_8 root. Pain may radiate down along the small-finger side of the arm and terminate in the little finger. Sensory changes may occur in the same area. Damage to this root causes weakness in the triceps, the muscles that raise and bend the wrist and fingers, and those that allow you to spread apart and bring together your fingers. The triceps reflex may be reduced.

These are typical but not absolute pain patterns. The same applies to the lumbar roots described below. Some people are wired a little differently.

Arm pain from a herniated cervical disk is common, usually occurring in thirty- to fifty-year-olds. Unlike lumbar disks, which usually herniate from lifting, carrying, or excessive bending (à la Mr. Peck), cervical disks are often herniated while we sleep.

Turning the head from side to side or sleeping on the stomach with the head turned to the side is a good position to herniate an already weakened cervical disk. This change in position in bed often occurs as we enter and leave the state of dream sleep. So we may awaken with a crick in our neck, which travels down an arm. Cervical-disk herniations may produce worse pain when a person carries or lifts on the side of the herniation, turns the head to the side, or strains or bears down through lifting a heavy load, coughing, sneezing, or having a bowel movement.

Bearing down makes all disk herniation pain at any spinal level worse because the pressure within the chest and abdomen increases during this type of effort and is transmitted to the inside of the disks. Any weakness within the annulus allows more disk material to herniate during increased pressure within the disk. In turn, more pressure may be exerted on a compromised spinal root, causing more pain.

Pain from cervical and lumbar herniations is typically reduced when you bend forward, thus opening the spinal canal and the foramina and thereby relieving the pressure on the root. Pain is worse when you bend backward. (These positions reduce and increase, respectively, pain from root pressure of stenosis and the narrowing of the spinal canal and foramina, too.) In any disk herniation causing root compression, you may experience throbbing pain like a toothache, pins and needles, or a burning sensation. The pain may be so severe that your back is locked in spasm, or it may be just a dull ache that increases with movement.

Thoracic Disks

The thoracic spine, behind the chest, is relatively safe from disk herniation because it hardly moves and is curved slightly backward, thus placing more pressure on the front of the disks. When these disks herniate, it is due to the weight on the thoracic spine from the body above the level of herniation or from a trauma, such as falling. A thoracic-disk herniation may cause pain radiating under the ribs, in the chest, upper abdomen, or around the thoracic spine and shoulder blades in the back of the body. Symptoms vary from a band of chest pain (the most common symptom), deep, dull pain behind the breastplate or stomach, or pain between the shoulder blades. Disk herniations of this type are not easily recognized by nonspecialists unfamiliar with this problem. They may go undiagnosed for a while, their symptoms often being confused with a heart, lung, gastrointestinal, or musculoskeletal problem.

Lumbar Disks

Any lumbar disk can rupture. The ones at the bottom of the spine herniate most frequently because they carry a greater proportion of the body's weight. Herniated lumbar disks can often be identified by the pattern of pain and nerve loss in the leg. The spinal cord does not extend below L_{1-2}. However, disk herniation in the lumbar spine that primarily affects the foramen—herniating off to the side of the spine—usually damages the exiting root at that level. Those that herniate centrally into the canal may damage the root that exits the spine one level below. This depends on the size of the canal in relation to the disk and the location of the herniation and the roots exiting the dural sac.

At the L_{3-4} level, a disk herniation may result in damage to the L_3 root exiting the spine, on the side of the disk, in the foramen, or the L_4 root off to one side in the canal. The same pattern applies to the other lumbar disks. The following patterns of pain, weakness, numbness, and reflex loss exist for various lumbar roots likely to be affected by disk herniations.

- Damage to the L_3 root results in pain to the front of the thigh to the inner part of the knee. Sensory changes, such as numbness and tingling, may occur in this area. Weakness may occur in the quadriceps (the muscle that straightens the knee) and the muscle that raises the thigh with the knee bent and the foot on the ground. There may be reduction of the knee reflex.

- If the L_4 root is damaged, it may result in pain along the nerve root that runs down the leg to the front of the ankle. Sensory changes may occur in the same area. Weakness of the quadriceps and reduction of the knee reflex may exist.

- The L_5 root, if damaged, results in pain that radiates down the leg, over the outside of the calf, and over the arch of the foot to the big toe. Muscles controlled by this root raise the foot and curl the big toe upward. Sensory changes may occur in the same area. There is no reflex loss with damage to this root.
- The S_1 nerve root can also be damaged, usually from a disk herniation at L_5–S_1. This causes pain that radiates down the leg into the back of the calf and the outside of the foot. This root, if damaged, causes weakness of the muscle that allows you to stand on your toes. Sensation may be altered in the same area as the pain. The ankle reflex may be reduced.

Characteristically, people with herniated lumbar disks have pain while bending, sitting, walking, and bearing down.

Sciatica Pain from Lumbar Disks

Sciatica is a term used to describe pain radiating along the route of the sciatic nerve, from the low back to the buttock and down the leg to the foot. This can occur from herniation, lumbar stenosis, spinal tumor, a torn annulus of a lower lumbar disk, damage to or irritation of the sciatic nerve in the buttock, myofascial pain emanating from the buttock muscles, or a painful sacroiliac joint. Sciatica from disk herniations occurs most commonly from a lumbar disk pressing on the L_4, L_5, and S_1 roots, all of which when compressed may radiate pain to the lower leg and foot. The sciatic nerve consists of the L_5, S_1, and S_2 roots.

Generally, leg pain from lumbar-disk herniations is worse when sitting and possibly standing and walking and less when lying in bed on the back with a pillow under the knees or, possibly, on the side. (Which side depends on where the herniation is and what makes you feel better.)

DIAGNOSING NERVE PAIN FROM DISK HERNIATION

Pain caused by irritation of a spinal root is radicular pain. As you've learned, many disk herniations can be clinically suspected by the pain symptoms in the spinal area—neck or lower back—and in the arm or leg. The amount of disk that is herniated, the severity of the pain and its associated neurological problems (weakness, numbness, or bowel or bladder difficulties), and the degree and length of disability contribute to choosing treatment.

An MRI can obtain images from inside the spinal canal and is the most sensitive test for identifying the location of a disk herniation and nerve compression. The MRI can also show where the extruded pieces of the disk went since they often migrate. Some herniated disks are enormous, others are tiny. Even enormous herniations do not always cause pain. Radicular pain, or nerve damage, only depends on whether the disk compresses a root. Some tiny disk fragments may cause symptoms just because they happen to be situated in such a way as to cause pressure on a root, one that is trapped between the small fragment in the front of the root, and a bony protuberance or enlarged ligament that extends into the spinal canal or foramen behind. The presence of the disk in front of the root forms a pincer or pliers that compresses the delicate nerve against the hard surface behind it.

If you cannot have an MRI because of a pacemaker or other metal in your body, a CT scan can be done. It is usually not as sensitive as an MRI, but it certainly can identify disk herniations. Annular tears, however, can be seen only on MRI.

An electromyogram (EMG) can confirm the clinical suspicion of nerve compression, but it won't identify the specific cause. There really is no reason for an EMG if the radiological tests show the cause of pain. Most EMGs used for evaluation of compressive spinal problems are unnecessary.

For more detailed information on these tests, go back to Chapter 3.

Conservative Treatment

Most people with herniated disks recover with rest, gradual mobilization, and pain medications. Anyone with progressive neurological dysfunction such as the sudden onset of bowel or bladder incontinence needs immediate surgical evaluation. These are rare conditions. Otherwise, pain-relieving medications (see below), local heat, massage, acupuncture, ultrasound, electric stimulation, and TENS (see Chapter 16), may all help reduce pain temporarily, giving the herniated disk a chance to shrink, which is how you get better. However, none of these therapies will heal the disk and permanently eliminate the pain it created.

The nucleus is about 90 percent water. Herniated nuclear fragments dry out and shrink. Also, the body recognizes disk material that is outside the annulus as foreign and tries to remove it. Specialized cells migrate to the site of the extrusion and digest it. This cellular activity is part of inflammation. As part of this process, the cleanup cells release enzymes that help break down the disk. However, these chemicals may also irritate the nearby spinal nerve root. *In 80 percent of patients with lumbar- and 70 percent of patients with cervical disk-herniations who experience pain and other symptoms, conservative or nonsurgical therapy works. Remember that!*

If symptoms have not begun to disappear over a month

(that doesn't mean they are completely gone), it may not be possible to wait longer before getting surgery. Many factors have to be considered, including your personality, lifestyle, professional commitments, general health, and history of spinal problems.

Medications

The drug therapy for a herniated disk consists of anti-inflammatory drugs, muscle relaxants, and narcotics. NSAIDs reduce the pain from inflammation around the root.

Corticosteroids (dexamethasone [Decadron], methyl-prednisolone [Medrol], prednisolone [Prednisone]) are many times more potent than NSAIDs. Nerves under pressure from disk herniations swell and press against the herniated disk, further increasing the pressure on the root. Theoretically, the steroids reduce the swelling in the compressed nerves, shrinking and reducing the pressure on them, with the result of reducing pain and deficit. They may be taken orally for a week or two for significant pain or injected as epidurals into the epidural space around the compressed root.

Oral steroids should be tried first for two weeks, repeated once if needed, before epidurals are considered, unless the oral steroids are ineffective, not well tolerated, or inadvisible. (They worsen ulcers, for example.) Oral or epidural corticosteroids may help reduce pain from root compression from disk herniations which are likely to go away over time. They do nothing to help the disk diminish in size, however. Therefore, it makes no sense to employ oral steroids or epidurals in the treatment of pain and deficits from chronic disk herniations, ones that are unlikely to disappear over time.

Corticosteroids often cause insomnia, but your doctor can prescribe Valium-like drugs to combat this and help sleep more soundly so that you don't toss and turn. With cervical-disk herniations, the use of such drugs makes it possible for you to sleep on your back, which minimizes pressure on the compressed root from turning your head to the side while lying on your stomach or side. I usually prescribe it to be taken a half hour before bedtime.

Epidurals are corticosteroids, sometimes combined with local anesthetics, that are injected into the epidural space. They may be repeated for a series of three or four over several weeks to a few months. Epidural administration of medications may be performed in the office blindly (without radiological guidance) or using a fluoroscopy unit or CT scanner. Using radiological guidance, the medication is injected into the epidural space through the foramen (for a disk affecting the root in the foramen) or between the lamina or bony arches in the back of the vertebra (for a more centrally located disk herniation). The more accurately the compressed root is covered with steroids, the more likely is the epidural to benefit the patient. I prefer using radiological guidance for all my procedures. Furthermore, since in the neck and thoracic spine the spinal cord is in jeopardy from incorrectly administered epidurals, radiological guidance should be used for epidural and other injections. (See Chapter 18 for more on oral and epidural steroids.)

Muscle relaxants relieve painful muscle spasm, a reflex spasm from underlying root irritation. The same root that connects nerves to the arm or leg muscles and skin also supplies the back muscles and skin. If it is irritated, it can result in increased tone in some of the muscles in the form of spasm.

Narcotics are effective in relieving moderate-to-severe pain. Narcotics may cause constipation, which increases the need to bear down during a bowel movement. This in turn may result in more pain and possibly increased disk herniation. A laxative regimen should be followed while on narcotics. This includes six to eight eight-ounce glasses of water daily, a high-fiber diet, Metamucil, two double-strength Senokot tablets every morning, and stool softeners (Colace three times daily). If this regimen is ineffective, Lactulose, a prescription syrup, may be prescribed.

All of the above drugs may be used simultaneously if needed to relieve severe radicular pain. Go to Chapter 17 for more explanation on how these drugs can help relieve pain.

Other drugs that may help relieve pain from compressed nerves include antiseizure medications, tricyclic antidepressants, and Valium-type drugs.

TREATING PAIN FROM CERVICAL-DISK HERNIATIONS

Most of the time, the pain from a herniated cervical disk can be controlled with rest, medication, and nonsurgical treatment. Once the pain ceases, it is unlikely to return; it may take longer for arm weakness and numbness to go away. Sometimes, the deficit following disk herniation never disappears completely, even though the pain subsides. A small degree of numbness or weakness may remain.

How to Wear a Cervical Collar

Wearing a soft cervical support collar for several weeks day and night helps rest your neck. After that, you can wear it intermittently for pain flare-ups or in situations where the neck can be jostled or turned excessively. The collar also reminds you not to turn your head too far in traffic. Of course, you must take that into consideration while driving and take necessary precautions. Your disk herniation can be made worse by a rear-end collision.

Sleeping on your back should rest the roots compressed by the disk. Have the collar properly fitted so that it is comfortable yet still supportive. It should close in the front, not the back, a contradiction of what most physicians and the people selling these collars say. The forward position is best accomplished by wearing the thick part of the collar behind the neck and the smaller part (where the closure is) in front of the neck. This posture of neck flexion, or bending the neck forward, opens the spinal canal and foramen, relieving root pressure from disk herniation.

Wearing the collar day and night for months may weaken your neck muscles somewhat. Be sure to talk with your doctor about long-term use.

Manual Traction

Theoretically, manual traction can help open up the cervical foramen where the nerve root exits the spinal canal. I think there is no basis for traction for any disk herniations unless there is a serious cervical spinal fracture. It is performed by strapping a device under the chin and behind the head, attaching it to a rope that is looped over a pulley, and having a weight at its other end. The patient sits in front of a door in the house. The pulley is attached to the door frame, and the weight causes the rope to pull the head of the patient on the other side of the pulley up and toward the ceiling. If this temporarily relieves the pain, a home treatment unit can be prescribed. This should only be done under supervision of a physical therapist, who can also prescribe exercises to relieve pressure on the nerve root.

Even if traction works, the effect is likely to be short-lived, only hours at best, until the disk recedes spontaneously or is removed surgically. I am adamantly opposed to chiropractic manipulation of the neck of anyone with a significant disk herniation. I have seen this type of treatment further herniate a previously herniated cervical disk, resulting in the need for urgent surgery. (I have nothing against gentle massage, which may be performed by chiropractors.)

TREATING PAIN FROM LUMBAR-DISK HERNIATIONS

Relief from pain caused by lumbar-disk herniation calls for conservative treatment, such as medication and rest as needed. You should get out of bed and ambulate as well as you can. Strict bed rest is no longer thought to be beneficial. If you wish to use anything else, like a lumbar support, do so if you think it makes you feel better. It isn't clear that these devices or others like them really do anything to make you heal, except reminding you not to bend too suddenly. Like the excessive use of a cervical collar, these supports, if used for extensive periods, such as over a span of months, may weaken your back.

Lying on your back with a pillow under your legs or resting on your side with a pillow placed between them removes tension from the inflamed nerve and reduces pressure on the herniated lumbar disk. As soon as possible, you should start walking on a flat surface. Stairs must be climbed with extreme care since the need to bear down while climbing stairs might exacerbate the disk herniation. Furthermore, if you have leg weakness from it, stair-climbing may prove difficult.

As the pain works out of the lower back and leg, various exercises help strengthen the low back and abdominal muscles to prevent recurrences (see Chapter 16).

LIFESTYLE CHANGES

Lifestyle changes can improve the quality of life following a disk herniation and possibly save you from surgery. Lifting, coughing, and other forms of straining are bad for any herniated disk, as these activities make the disk bulge out more thus further pressing on the root, worsening the pain, and increasing the possible need for surgery. With a fresh disk herniation, don't lift anything (including your baby or a purse weighing more than a pound). Take cough medicine if necessary. Use antihistamines if you sneeze from allergies. Use stool softeners to avoid straining during bowel movements.

If you are overweight, losing weight in the long run should reduce the wear on your lumbar disks, supporting spinal ligaments, and, for that matter, weight-bearing joints in the lower limbs. (Losing weight also reduces the risk of developing diabetes and reduces blood pressure.) With or without a genetic curse, most people's obesity results from eating the wrong types of food and eating more calories than they burn.

You cannot really prevent your disks from wearing out, but you can take steps to lower your risk of damaging them (see Chapter 21).

SURGERY FOR DISK HERNIATION

Discectomy, foramenotomy and, in the neck, anterior decompression and fusion (ACDF) are all operations that may be used to treat problems from a disk's pressing a nerve root. You will find the details of surgery in Chapter 19.

Surgery is sometimes indicated to decompress a root pressed between a disk and a piece of bone or ligament or to remove the portion of the disk that is pressing on the nerve. In general, the larger the disk herniation, the greater the pain and disability, the more likelihood of significant weakness or numbness, and the lack of beneficial response to a few weeks of conservative care all increase the likelihood that surgery is needed. However, indications for surgery are not always clear-cut, making the decision difficult for many people. For the rare person with the loss of bladder or bowel function (cauda equina syndrome) from a large disk herniation, emergency surgery is the only choice. Similarly, serious signs of spinal cord compression from disk herniation require prompt surgical decompression.

Certain types of muscle weakness may also lead to early surgery. If your foot is in a dropped position and cannot be raised off the floor, early surgical intervention must be considered. While you may recover from this situation without it, it may take some time. Any permanent residual weakness of this sort may make walking difficult for the rest of your life.

Factors that play a role in the decision include your pain tolerance, emotional response, work demands, and other lifestyle issues.

Remember the following statement that applies to the vast majority of people with back pain: *Disk surgery should be done primarily for the relief of radicular leg, arm, or shoulder pain and weakness or numbness in the leg, arm, or shoulder. As a rule, it should not be performed for the relief of neck or back pain alone.* Surgery should not be taken lightly. No matter what technique is used, the spine and surrounding ligaments are permanently damaged and weakened by surgery. Sometimes, the risk of future surgery is increased. At least 10 percent of discectomy patients undergo further spine surgery.

Surgery does help to eliminate the symptoms of sciatica more quickly than conservative—nonsurgical—treatment. However, one study indicates that if you are willing to wait it out and undergo nonsurgical treatment, by ten years following the onset of sciatica, there will be no difference in outcome between patients who had surgery and those who did not. My clinical experience does not support the conclusion of this report, but even if the conclusion is true, only you can decide how long—weeks, months, or years—you can live in pain or on chronic pain medication instead of proceeding with disk surgery. Unlike with a growing malignant tumor or blocked coronary arteries in need of a stent, you won't die from a disk herniation if the surgery to treat it is delayed. However, the pain and, perhaps worse, the weakness or numbness from a disk herniation compressing a root is another matter. Tolerance for pain and the ability to live with loss of neurological function depends on a host of factors. Pain from most herniated disks often goes away on its own, and so does any minor weakness and numbness accompanying them.

One study compared 166 sciatica patients who were treated with laminectomy with 417 others who were treated with only bed rest and a back brace. The study showed that 97 percent of the surgical patients had good results after one month compared with 76 percent of the bed rest group. At six months however, 99 percent of the group that had undergone the surgery reported good results, and so did 93 percent of the bed rest group. I'm not suggesting that you stay in bed for six months or that you use a brace for that time. But this study illustrates the value of deferring surgery, if possible, for four to eight weeks. The problems from many disk herniations will improve in that time. However, also keep in mind that as a rule, patients with disk herniations causing significant root compression that results in severe pain and especially in significant weakness or numbness do *not* improve in a timely fashion with conservative treatment alone.

Key Points about Back Pain from Disk Herniations

- Most disk herniations occur at spinal segments that are maximally bent forward: the lower neck and lumbar spine.

- A lower lumbar-disk herniation may cause true nerve root pain, commonly called sciatica.
- An MRI can obtain images from inside the spinal canal and foramen and is the most sensitive test for identifying the location of a disk herniation and nerve compression.
- Most people with herniated disks recover with rest, gradual mobilization, pain medications, and, sometimes, physical therapy or epidural steroid injections.
- Progressive or sudden onset of neurological problems or bowel or bladder problems may require surgical intervention.
- After a disk herniation, changes in lifestyle may save you from surgery.

Chapter 10

Discogenic Back Pain

When the annulus—the cover around the disk—tears, pain may occur. The annulus has nerve fibers, unlike the nucleus. When a tear occurs in the annulus, you may feel pain in the neck or lower back and areas overlying and around the tear. Pain may also travel down the arm or leg, as with a true disk herniation.

Chemicals irritating to nerves are produced inside degenerating disks, those which are candidates for annular tears or herniations. Once there is an annular tear, these noxious substances may leak out through it and irritate the nearby spinal roots. The brain cannot tell if the pain is from disk herniation, which irritates the root by pressure, or a chemically irritated root.

Although an annular tear may produce pain that is referred or travels from the neck to an arm or from the lower back to a leg, it can never produce weakness or numbness. Only compression of the root can do that. (All disk herniations are accompanied by annular tears but not all annular tears are associated with disk herniations.) Annular tears usually heal in two to three months. However, they can tear again and cause pain again. This phenomenon is part of chronic discogenic pain. Discogenic pain, to the extent it is understood, arises from abnormalities within the disk itself and has nothing to do with pain from a herniation, which occurs as a result of root compression by the herniated disk.

DIAGNOSING DISCOGENIC PAIN

A discogram can confirm or eliminate nonherniated disks as sources of pain. If an MRI shows a tear in the annulus or disk covering, usually coupled with other signs of disk degeneration, a discogram may determine if that disk and nearby ones are a cause of pain (see Chapter 3).

CONSERVATIVE TREATMENT OF DISCOGENIC PAIN

Most people with annular tears recover with rest, pain medications, and a gradual resumption of normal activity. NSAIDs, muscle relaxants for spasm, and narcotics should be used as needed. Sometimes physical therapy or epidural steroid injections may be used. Local heat, massage, acupuncture, ultrasound, electric stimulation, and TENS (see Chapter 16) may all help reduce pain temporarily while the annulus heals. However, none of these therapies will heal the disk and permanently reduce the pain it created.

Most discogenic pain comes from an annular tear, although that may not be the whole story. Although there is no pressure on a spinal root in this condition, it does hurt. Activity reduction and lifestyle modification so as not to bear down—risking a further tear or a disk herniation through the tear—is important.

The vast majority of annular tears causing discogenic pain heal without difficulty. For those that don't, there are several minimally interventional treatments presented below. Also, discogenic pain is one of the leading reasons for lumbar fusions in the United States—usually an inappropriate reason for this surgery, as you will see later.

Epidural Steroid Injections

Besides acting on the swollen, inflamed nerves, the liquid in the steroid epidural injection also flushes away the chemicals produced by the annular tears that cause root inflammation and pain. Studies on epidurals show that they work well for a very small specific group of people, such as those under forty who have not previously had surgery or those with pain lasting less than three months. If used at all, epidural injections are most appropriate as a short-term treatment for those whose spine-related pain also travels or radiates down a leg or arm. They are not helpful for localized neck or back pain unaccompanied by leg or arm pain. (See Chapter 18 for more information about this therapy technique.) In theory, epidurals in the neck and thoracic area risk damaging the spinal cord. In practice, this occurs rarely. However, the risks and costs of epidurals are real enough that they should not be considered in the same light as taking Tylenol.

Intradiskal Therapy

To understand this kind of therapy, you must understand the theory behind discogenic pain. Yes, annular tears cause pain. However, many people have annular tears that appear as incidental findings on MRIs obtained for pain distant from the tear. For example, a disk herniation may exist, thus explaining a sciatica-like leg pain. However, on the same MRI, an annular tear at L_{2-3}, six inches above L_5–S_1, may also exist, which has seemingly nothing to do with your very low back and sciatica-like leg pain. Everyone with discogenic pain has disk degeneration and annular tears but not everyone with disk degeneration and annular tears has discogenic pain. There is far more to discogenic pain than disk degeneration, but it is not clear why some degenerated, torn disks hurt and others do not. Nor is it clear why most acutely painful degenerated disks, with annular tears become less painful in two to three months while in others, the pain persists.

To understand the therapy of discogenic pain, you must first understand how the pain from painful disks is transmitted to the brain. The treatment of discogenic pain is analogous to treating painful facets with radiofrequency lesions. With painful facets, we may not know why they hurt or be able to stop facet degeneration—to the extent that it causes pain—but we can control facet-related pain by cutting nerves, the lines of communication from painful facets to the brain.

As disks degenerate, they crack in both the annulus and the nucleus. The nucleus, you recall, has no nerves in it; the annulus does. In degenerated disks, nerves from the annulus grow into the nucleus along these cracks. In those patients with degenerated disks that hurt, that have discogenic pain, these nerves may have something to do with the propagation of pain from the nucleus and annulus. Your body weight increases intradiskal pressure while standing, causing pain in predisposed, degenerated disks. Even while you are lying down, rotational and bending forces on the degenerated disk may result in pain.

Discograms increase internal pressure on a disk. For those disks that hurt, reproducing everyday forces that increase intradiskal pressure causes pain. Partial destruction of these nerves within the nucleus and, possibly, those at the interior of the annulus may relieve discogenic pain. The various minimally invasive treatments for discogenic pain all involve inserting a probe into a painful disk and heating its interior. There are different theories on why these treatments are effective; I believe it is the lesioning of intradiskal nerves that relieve the pain.

Laser and Other Therapies

Laser therapy, according to some studies, is an effective therapy for lumbar discogenic pain. Radiofrequency lesioning can be delivered right into the disk's nucleus to relieve pain. A newer therapy called IDET (intradiskal electrothermal lysis) uses conductive heat. It became very popular several years ago. These therapies are explained in detail in Chapter 18.

WHEN TO CONSIDER SURGERY

Two surgical remedies have been touted for discogenic pain. The newer one is disk replacement surgery. Unfortunately, this replacement is best performed just as disks are beginning to degenerate, before the spine around the disk also wears down, in young people with little complaints about their spines. Furthermore, the operation to replace the disks requires extensive surgery, and the disk replacements are highly experimental. If they break down, what is the next step: another disk replacement or a fusion of the vertebral bodies around the worn-down disk? I would certainly never send anyone for such surgery in the foreseeable future.

As yet there is no good information on the results of artificial disk implantation, including how they hold up over time. Moreover, the surgical procedure to remove your painful disk and put in a new one is an enormous undertaking.

Half of lumbar fusions in the United States are performed for disk herniations or discogenic pain. Using fusion for a simple disk herniation or discogenic pain is akin to killing a rabbit with a cannon when a small rifle will do. Fusion surgery for the majority of disk herniations may resolve the problem automatically: The disk is removed from the root at the time of the fusion. However, a simpler discectomy is usually sufficient. Fusions are useful only if the spine is unstable in the area of the disk in question, that is, one vertebra wiggles over another. In discogenic pain, fusion is not only extraordinary surgical excess; it is also likely not to achieve its objection, the reduction of back pain. Indeed, it is very likely to cause chronic postoperative pain, perhaps different from and as bad as, if not worse than, the pain before surgery. A third of patients who have undergone lumbar fusions live in chronic pain and disability; 30 to 70 percent do not return to work. Moreover, no high-quality academic studies support this surgical treatment of discogenic pain or compare it to the other less-invasive therapies described above. As a treatment for back pain not due to severe instability with compression of the nerve roots, fusion is usually unsuccessful in achieving the objective of lessening a patient's pain. There *is* a clear role for fusions in pain and neurological dysfunction from spinal instability, as you will see in Chapter 11.

There is little if any role for fusions in the treatment of most discogenic pain. Indeed, I tell my patients with discogenic pain: "If I can't significantly diminish your pain through procedures, we'll have to find some medication regimen and lifestyle modification to permanently maintain you. Do not have a fusion. If you do, you'll still permanently need chronic medication and lifestyle modification." I have this opinion because in hundreds of patients, I have never really failed in my attempts to treat discogenic pain. All of my patients with this problem obtained sufficient relief from my ministrations that they stayed at or returned to work. However, I have many disabled patients who have had fusions before they came to my practice. They obviously see me because they are in severe pain.

Key Points about Discogenic Pain

- Discogenic pain arises from abnormalities within the disk itself. It has nothing to do with pain from a herniation, which occurs as a result of root compression by the herniated disk.
- Most people with discogenic pain recover with rest, pain-relieving medications, and other conservative treatment.
- Epidural injections work well for short-term relief on some people with this type of pain.
- Radiofrequency lesioning of the disk and other techniques, such as IDET, are helpful therapy for longer-term relief.
- Well-controlled academic studies are required to truly evaluate the various therapies for discogenic pain.
- Contemplating having an artificial disk is premature.
- There is no need for surgery for most discogenic pain.

Chapter 11

Spinal Slippage and Instability: Spondylolisthesis and Spondylolysis

Spondylolisthesis (spon-dee-lo-lies-THEESIS) is an age-related degeneration of moving parts of the spine (disks, facets, ligaments) that causes slippage and instability between vertebrae. This means that one vertebra has slipped out of line with the one above or below. Slippage may vary in degree. In some people, it may not cause much instability; in others it may be quite unstable and slip back and forth whenever the spine moves. Slippage of one body over another may occur forward or backward. Sideways and rotational slippage may also occur in people with scoliosis. Unstable vertebrae are wiggling bones that may bang into the nerve roots within the canal or foramen, the windows through which nerves exit the spine. In turn, this causes intermittent or continuous pain and possibly weakness or numbness.

Curiously, over time, elderly people with degenerated spines often remain stable despite the slippage earlier in life. Degenerative changes in aging spines create spinal narrowing (stenosis), which actually limits further instability. Disks dry out and lose their height, so previously slipped vertebrae come closer together. Calcified and hardened ligaments and facet joints also help stabilize the vertebrae.

Unstable slippage is more often seen in younger people, who still have well-preserved unflattened disks that provide a large wiggling space between loose, slipped vertebrae.

The degree of slippage and instability and the amount of pressure on nerve roots influences the need for and choice of treatment needed to relieve pain or neurological dysfunction. Relatively stable and previously slipped spines with a narrowed spinal canal and compressed nerve roots may require surgical decompression with laminotomy or foramenotomy. Patients with a high degree of instability and slippage may also need fusion.

We are all born with different genetics, which partially explains the variability in disease among us. Some people have lumbar facets that are more likely to keep the spine stable than others do. Some are born with vertebra whose bony arches don't join properly. (Think of the variation in shapes of noses, finger joints, and other small bones.) Cartilage plates allow for the growth of bone while we are young. Such plates exist in the lamina of the vertebrae between the facets. Before birth, our bones become solid, and these cartilage plates usually close. When they do not, there is no union of the bony arches, and a condition called spondylolysis results. This occurs at L_5. The normally stabilizing facets at the side of the arch are no longer connected to the vertebra. This can happen on one side or, more commonly, on both sides of the L_5 vertebra. If you have such anatomy, you are more likely to have a spinal slippage of L_5 than someone without spondylolysis.

Genetics and environment play a role in spinal degeneration. Some people have good spines, others begin to have problems in their twenties. By the time they are fifty, their spines appears to be those of eighty-year-olds. The degenerating system no longer holds the vertebrae tightly in place, so they slip around. On the other hand, lifestyle can damage your spine. The more you use your neck in such an activity as wrestling or neck and lower spine in manual labor or playing football, the more likely you are to wear them out, indeed accelerate the degenerative process. Wearing the spine out in these ways are environmental and therefore preventable. However, whether you engage in such activities or not, there is still your genetics, which influences the rate of decline of your spine. We can do little about our genetic inheritance.

As the body reacts to excessive wear, the ligaments inside the spine—ligamenta flava—bulge inside the epidural space and later calcify. Once the calcification of these ligaments and the facets occurs, the slipping spine stabilizes. In the

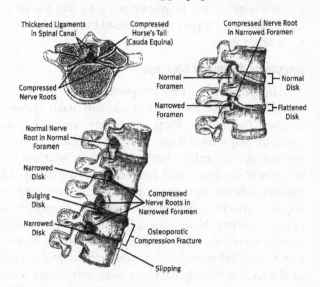

FIGURE 9. Diseased lumbar spine in aging; showing slippage, narrowing of the spinal canal and foramen, and an osteoporotic fracture.

meantime, the disks degenerate; later, the bulging calcified ligamenta flava and arthritic facets fill up the epidural space and foramen, compressing the nerves there. This arthritic narrowing of the spinal cavity and foramen is called stenosis. (See next chapter.) The slippage of the vertebra is called spondylolisthesis. As it is part of the aging process, it is referred to as degenerative spondylolisthesis.

Lumbar Slippage

The most common site for spondylolisthesis is L_4 on L_5 in the lower back, also a common site for lumbar wear and tear, as evidenced by the many disk herniations and later narrowing of the canal or stenosis at that level. The slippage typically occurs in patients with degenerated disks. Slippage occurs somewhat less frequently at L_3–L_4 and less so at L_5–S_1. At L_5–S_1 slippage may be caused by spondylolysis of L_5, as noted above.

Symptoms of Lumbar Slippage

Many people never have symptoms or pain with either spondylolysis (lysis for short) or relatively stable spondylolisthesis (listhesis for short). Others may have much more pain with only a small degree of spinal instability. The reason for this is unclear, but it depends in part on the anatomy of the spinal canal and foramen. Small canals and foramen, whether from the genetics you are born with or acquired arthritic calcification, allow less slippage than open ones before the vertebra or ligament slams on and off a tender nerve root, causing pain in a leg. When you do have pain, it may feel much like a muscle strain in the low back or like sciatica. Initially, pain may occur only during activity, or it may become constant and even interfere with sleep. Unstable spines slip when you are lying down. Truly unstable spines are often painful and far more often require fusion surgery than minimal slippage, which is relatively stable. The size of the interior of the spine is also important in this determination.

Here are the most common symptoms of painful, grossly unstable lumbar spondylolisthesis:

- low-back aching pain that feels much like a muscle strain
- less pain while you sit than when you stand
- spasms that stiffen the back and tighten the hamstring muscles in the back of the thigh
- occasional pain radiating down one or both legs (from pressure on the roots within the spinal canal or the neural foramen)
- pain during activity that progresses through the day and even interferes with sleep
- pain that increases when you bend backward, lessens when you bend forward

Cervical Slippage

Extremely rarely slippage can occur in the neck, sometimes causing severe pain and requiring surgery. The vertebrae in the neck are smaller, and so is the spinal canal, so they can tolerate far less pressure than the nerve roots in the lumbar spine. Severe pressure here is more likely to cause permanent damage. Arthritic deposits and disk herniations in the neck can cause severe cord and root compression, so even minor slippage may further narrow the canal and foramen. This can cause pain, weakness, numbness, and bowel and bladder problems, depending on whether the cord or simply the roots are pinched. If cervical spinal cord compression causes weakness in the legs as well as arms and makes walking difficult, the pressure must be surgically removed to prevent permanent neurological damage. Small slippages within the cervical spine that do not cause pain or neurological problems can be helped with exercise; they do not need surgery. However, they should be watched for increase in symptoms or pain.

DIAGNOSING SPINAL SLIPPAGE AND OTHER PROBLEMS

Some physicians erroneously feel that spinal problems can be diagnosed with a clinical examination. Even the best clinical evaluation must be confirmed or modified after obtaining high-quality radiological studies. In an exam, a doctor may ask you to stand, then gently lean backward and toward the side that is in pain or straight back if the pain affects both sides. If this brings on your usual back pain, there may be slippage. But so may sore muscles, painful facets, a torn annulus, spondylolysis, a vertebra invaded by tumor, or a small disk herniation: alone, in various combinations, or possibly with spondylolisthesis. In other words, it is impossible to make an absolute diagnosis based solely on your complaints and a physical examination. The side view of your spine in X-rays and CT and MRI scans will show the position of the vertebrae and whether there is spondylolisthesis.

Spondylolisthesis is graded, based on X-ray results:

> **Grade I** is less than 25 percent slippage of one
>   vertebra on top of another
> **Grade II** is 25 percent to 50 percent slippage
> **Grade III** is 50 percent to 75 percent slippage
> **Grade IV** is more than 75 percent slippage.

Side view X-rays and CT scans are best for revealing lysis. Spinal instability can be diagnosed only by flexion-extension views: X-rays taken while you bend forward (flex) and backward (extend).

TREATING SPONDYLOLYSIS AND SPINAL SLIPPAGE

Spondylolysis is irrelevant unless it causes slippage that results in pain and other symptoms. The diagnosis is made with flexion-extension X-rays, CT scans, and MRIs. For mild-to-moderate back pain from slippage, one should rest and refrain from the pain-producing activity.

Anti-inflammatory medicines, such as ibuprofen, may reduce back pain. If needed, mild-to-moderate strength narcotics, such as acetaminophen with codeine (Tylenol No. 3), acetaminophen with hydrocodone (Vicodin or Lortabs, for example), or acetaminophen with oxycodone (Percocet or Exocet) may be prescribed with good results. Oral corticosteroids can be used for this condition if there is leg pain from nerve root irritation. Similarly, epidurals and root blocks with corticosteroids may give temporary relief of root pain.

Nonsurgical therapy that may help includes:

- gentle physical therapy to strengthen back muscles and learn new ways to lift and bend
- hydrotherapy
- wearing a brace
- correcting posture

If the back pain does not respond to conservative treatment or signs of leg weakness and numbness develop, you need a CT/myelogram with flexion-extension views (bending forward and bending backward) to monitor the spinal anatomy under the stress of movement and determine the effect of spinal movement on compression of the nerve roots in the spinal canal or foramen.

The findings of these studies may prompt surgery to alleviate nerve root pressure from arthritic narrowing (stenosis), disk herniations or bulges, or a significantly unstable spine, which continually whacks the nerve roots as it slips. Significant instability requires fusion surgery (see Chapter 19).

Treatment for less significant instability depends on these factors:

- the anatomy the patient was born with (a narrow spinal canal), the severity and anatomy of their degenerative spinal problems (height of disks, vertical size of foramen, size of disk herniations, degree of acquired stenosis)
- tolerance for pain
- the ability to benefit from and tolerate pain medication
- lifestyle demands
- the imagination, judgment, and skill of the treating physicians and surgeons

Some of these patients can go for years without surgery by using pain medication and limiting their lifestyle.

Avoid surgery—including fusion—if you:

- have back pain in a stable spine or pain with minor instability
- have no disk herniations, or narrowing of the canal or foramen that cause leg pain because of root compression

Instead, use the full gamut of treatment available from the best physicians who specialize in managing this kind of low-back pain before considering fusion to stabilize your spine. You may have chronic pain after a fusion that is more severe than the pain from the slight spinal instability.

For more complicated spinal problems from instability you may need surgical decompression (the opening of a tight spine or removal of disks pressing on nerves) and in some cases fusion, to relieve symptoms.

See Chapter 19 for a full description of the types of surgery.

Before You Decide on Surgery

Before you go down the one-way road to surgery, including fusion, investigate all other means of treatment. There are ways to avoid surgery if you have low-grade slippage and instability with mild-to-moderate back or leg pain.

- Some people have abnormal movement of the spine when standing. They feel better in a forward, flexed posture. This may help take pressure off the squeezed roots in the canal or foramen.
- Limit heavy lifting: The strain from this activity could cause your spine to slip more.
- Analgesic medication may help chronic pain.
- Physical therapeutic treatments, such as strengthening exercises or wearing a brace, may help though usually not enough over a long period.
- Acupuncture, TENS, and gentle chiropractic manipulation may all be tried, though there will usually be little success. Theoretically, vigorous chiropractic manipulation can further destabilize some patients.

- Oral or injected steroids, including epidurals, may give temporary relief for a condition that will not improve.
- Radiofrequency lesions of the facets, treatments for discogenic pain, and other pain-relieving interventions don't solve this problem.

If a conservative approach does not sufficiently relieve pain or surrenders too much of lifestyle, find a skilled experienced surgeon who is willing to try to consider decompressing you without fusion if your listhesis is low grade and relatively stable. This depends on the surgeon's skill and judgment and your anatomy. You should also understand that if you are one of the approximately 15 percent of stable listhesis patients who do become unstable after a simple decompression, you may require a fusion in the future. For those with significantly unstable slippage, surgical decompression should include fusion, since the instability will worsen after simple decompression.

SURGERY

Back pain, with or without leg pain, occurs as spinal degeneration progresses. If there is leg pain, your body is clearly telling you that the nerve roots are being pinched by disk herniations, bulging calcified ligaments and facets, or spinal slippage. Even if no roots are seriously compressed in a young unstable spine, gross instability pulls and pushes on the ligaments supporting the spine and the capsules of the facets, causing back pain, if nothing else.

Painful instability, even in the absence of disk herniations or stenosis, often requires surgical fusion in the long run, especially if roots are being compressed. For those with slippage and the other conditions mentioned, an otherwise straightforward disk operation or decompression of stenosis often will call for a fusion of the unstable vertebrae at the same time.

If you have disk herniations or stenosis and a relatively stable slippage, can your pain and dysfunction be relieved without resorting to a fusion? This is a very important question for you to ask your doctor. Every year there are thousands of patients with this complicated spinal picture who undergo fusions along with their decompressive surgery. To relieve them of their symptoms, reduce their need for analgesic medication, and increase the quality of their existence, they certainly need decompressive surgery. But do they need fusion?

Do You Need Fusion?

Your spine is stabilized by two facets, the intervertebral disks and the supporting ligaments. A simple decompressive laminotomy (removal of part of the bony arch in the back of the vertebra), laminectomy (removal of all of the arch), and even a partial removal of the facet joint (facetectomy) or opening of the bony window through which the root passes between the vertebral bodies behind the disk (foramenotomy) may be performed without further destabilizing the spine. (See Chapters 12 and 19.) If too much of the facet is removed in order to remove some disks herniated into the foramen or to remove pressure on a root from stenosis, the spine can become unstable.

Destabilization may be more likely to occur if both facets are partially removed and a laminectomy—rather than a laminotomy—is performed in decompressive surgery for stenosis. A laminectomy removes the supporting ligaments behind the vertebra; laminotomy preserves them. Some elegant surgeons minimize the risk of further spinal slippage after decompressive surgery without fusion by leaving in as much facet as possible or even decompressing both sides of a narrow canal through a simple one-sided laminotomy.

Most patients without preexisting slippage do not become unstable after routine spinal decompression for stenosis if the outermost part of the facet is left intact and the bony connection of the facet to the vertebra is not broken during surgery. However, the risk of instability increases in any operation on a spine with preexisting slippage. The greater the slippage and the more facet that must be shaved off to decompress the roots, the greater the risk of creating instability and further slippage. Leaving facets relatively intact to minimize further slippage while not adequately opening the sides of the canal and the foramen is also not a solution. After such excessively conservative surgery, you will still have ongoing leg pain and possibly weakness, and numbness.

Disk surgery with a laminotomy, for example, usually involves one side, so in theory it is less likely to destabilize an already slightly unstable spinal segment than two-sided decompressive surgery. However, a large, well-preserved disk in a scantily arthritic spinal segment (regardless of the patient's age) between two slipped but stable vertebrae increases the likelihood of instability over time or after, for example, a simple discectomy. Compare this with a slightly slipped but still mostly stable segment that is stabilized by a flat degenerated disk, arthritis in the facets, and calcium deposits (osteophytes) around the disk and nearby ligaments. This arthritic segment is already naturally semifused so is less likely to become unstable, even after surgery, than the more youthful segment described above.

Disk herniations in people with relatively well preserved disks and obvious spinal instability at the level of the herniation may have to consider having fusion along with a discectomy. Nevertheless, a simple discectomy without fusion may work well for some. This depends on the degree of instability, the site of the disk, size and location of its herniated portion, whether the patient had prior surgery at that location, and the skill of the surgeon. You should avoid a fusion for as long as possible.

In treating stenosis and minimizing the need for fusion, surgical judgment and skill are both of paramount importance in deciding how much bone and ligament to remove to provide adequate relief from whatever symptoms and nerve damage that exist. They are also key in determining who may be treated without fusion—a small risk of instability after surgery—and who must be fused at the time of decompression. A highly skilled surgeon can decompress a narrowed spinal segment (L_{4-5}, for example) in an older adult with a preexisting stable grade I slippage in the absence of a lysis with only about a 15 percent risk of destabilizing that segment of the spine.

Unfortunately, if you are like the older stenosis patient described above, the majority of surgeons in the United States today will want to combine decompression with fusion. There are several reasons for this. First, most surgeons though competent are not excellent. This is not meant to disparage them. The same applies to any occupation. Second, decompressing a complicated spine without causing instability takes time, but the modern insurance system pays a physician for neither time nor outcome. For the surgeon, it is about twice as lucrative to aggressively decompress the spine—widely open the spine and drill away most of the facets—thus making it unstable and then fuse the segment than it is to delicately decompress a segment and preserve its stability so that fusion is not required.

Find a conservative neurosurgeon or spine surgeon who will treat you with the least possible amount of surgery. Unnecessary fusions may not cost you anything out of pocket, but they may condemn you to chronic pain, frequent visits to the pain clinic, and possibly more surgery. And remember, once you have a fusion, it can't be undone. All too often there is no divorce from spinal surgery that created a chronically painful condition.

Key Points about Spondylolisthesis and Spondylolysis

- Spondylolysis has no significance unless there is also disk herniation, stenosis, or spondylolisthesis (or slippage) in a spine requiring surgery, at which point it may increase the risk of slippage.
- Spondylolisthesis occurs when one vertebra slips over another. It is a degenerative condition that occurs as you age.
- It is impossible to make an absolute diagnosis of spondylolisthesis without taking X-rays, CT scans, or MRIs to show the position of the vertebrae.
- Conservative treatment can ease pain from this condition.
- Spondylolisthesis, especially combined with stenosis or a disk herniation, may require surgery, but simple decompression of the spine *without* fusion should be considered whenever possible.
- Fusion usually is required to treat cases of significant pain due to nerve root compression in unstable spines.
- Fusion rarely may be required to treat cases of severe low back pain without root compression, but due to instability, not adequately controlled by lifestyle changes and potent pain relievers.
- In general, fusion for low back pain alone caused by instability should be used as a last choice. Back pain following fusion may be as bad as or worse than that from the instability before the fusion.

Chapter 12

Spinal-Canal Narrowing: Stenosis

Spinal stenosis is a narrowing of the spinal canal and sometimes the foramen. About 10 percent of people are born with narrow spinal canals, a problem called congenital stenosis. They are more likely to have problems with their spines than those with large canals. A small disk herniation in someone with a small canal is more likely to compress a nerve root than a similar herniation in someone with a large canal. Minor instability in a patient with a stenotic canal is more likely to cause nerve root irritation than in someone with a large canal. As the spinal canal narrows with age, a person born with an already narrow canal is likely to have pain earlier than someone born with a large canal.

Spondylosis (spon-dee-LOSIS) is an acquired form of spinal canal and, often, foramenal narrowing. Most patients and doctors call it stenosis so we'll do that, too. It is a slowly evolving process that takes years to develop. As it progresses, it may cause leg, arm, and back or neck pain, weakness, numbness, and difficulty in walking, especially long distances. It may result in bowel and bladder dysfunction if the spinal cord is compressed by severe cervical spinal canal narrowing. (Spondylosis or stenosis should not be confused with spondylolysis [a birth defect] and spondylolisthesis [slippage]; covered in the previous chapter.)

Theoretically, the processes that lead to acquired stenosis start in the late twenties as the disks, which are 90 percent water, dry out and lose volume. They also lose height, bringing the vertebra closer together. Unlike disk herniations, which usually improve without surgery, spondylosis, or acquired narrowing of the canal and foramen is a chronic condition that progressively gets worse. By the time most people have back pain or other symptoms, the narrowing is usually quite advanced.

These degenerating disks may become painful or herniated, and they also tend to bulge into the spinal canal and nearby foramen. Eventually, over years, these bulging disks become hardened with calcium deposits (calcify) The initial loss in height of the disks results in a slight slippage of one vertebra over another, thus putting increased pressure on the facets.

The yellow ligaments (ligamenta flava) that help stabilize the spine thicken and become stronger to accommodate the slightly unstable spine. These thickened ligaments compress the canal and foramen; eventually, they calcify, too. At the same time, the facets wear down and become arthritic and possibly painful. They develop calcium deposits that bulge outside as well as inside the spine, where they also compress the canal and foramen. These protuberant calcified deposits of facets and ligaments are called osteophytes.

The narrowing develops because all those calcified parts gradually become pincers within the canal and foramen. Not everyone with spinal narrowing has all the components of this pincer system, but if you have symptoms from stenosis, you have enough of a developed pincer to compress your nerve roots. Or if it occurs in the cervical and thoracic areas, it may compress your spinal cord as well as nerve roots. The pain of stenosis can be relieved for a long time with medication and changes in physical activity, but most people eventually need surgery to decompress the roots compressed by tight areas of the spine.

LUMBAR SPINAL STENOSIS

By far the most common area of the spine to develop acquired narrowing (spondylosis) is the lumbar spine, canal, and foramen. It may cause these symptoms:

- back pain
- radiating pain to one or both buttocks, the groin, hips, legs, and feet
- possible weakness and numbness in one or both legs

These problems may worsen with walking and, in severe cases, standing. Back and leg pain, weakness, and numbness may contribute to a bent-over posture and abnormal walking. Such symptoms are called neurogenic claudication: exercise-related pain and dysfunction from nerve root compression. There are two major explanations for the pain and dysfunction of lumbar stenosis.

First, the erect position increases the narrowing of the stenotic spinal canal—that pincer movement—by forcing the calcified already thickened ligamenta flava in the back and sides of the canal to further bulge into the canal, increasing the stenosis. In mild-to-moderate stenosis, forward bending of the spine opens the canal by reducing the internal bulging of the ligamenta flava into the canal. This relieves pressure on the nerves in the narrow areas of the canal. In severe stenosis, however, the spinal canal remains narrow regardless of posture, which is why many people with severe stenosis have pain, numbness, and weakness even in bed.

Second, circulatory disturbances may also play a part in the symptoms of stenosis. Here's one widely held theory. As you exercise, the heart pumps more blood. This supplies the muscles in use and also dilates the veins in the epidural space. In the stenotic portion of this space, these dilated veins further increase the pressure on the nerves, causing more pain and sometimes numbness, tingling, and even weakness of the legs. If you stop walking and sit in a slightly bent position for a minute or so, the pain and other symptoms are quickly relieved because the spine opens. This and the reduced necessity of the heart's pumping blood to muscles that are now resting allows the dilated veins to shrink. The whole process starts over again if you get up and walk.

Another theory is that the tight spine simply impairs circulation of blood to and from the compressed nerve roots. As these structures do more work—sending signals to and from the spinal cord providing you with the power and coordination to stand or walk—they require more blood. If they can't get what they need, they generate pain impulses and work inefficiently, resulting in weakness and numbness. When you sit and bend forward, the canal opens and blood supply is restored to the nerves, allowing them to catch up on their nutritional requirements. Your symptoms disappear until you walk or stand again.

Here's an example. When standing, Tim had increasing pain in his right back, thigh, and knee, which was relieved when he sat down. He rode his bicycle on a flat rural road several miles three times a week with no significant pain. But if he danced with his wife, his turn on the floor lasted only ten to fifteen minutes because of pain in his back and leg. Naturally, his wife didn't understand how he could ride his bicycle for hours on end but could not dance for more than ten minutes. Biking and dancing both require increased blood supply from the heart and result in dilated epidural veins. But Tim rode his bicycle, he was bent forward, a position that lessens spinal stenosis; when he danced, he was erect, an extended posture that increases the symptoms of spinal stenosis.

The pain of lumbar stenosis can be controlled for years with medication, including narcotics, and modification of exercise, such as walking less. But if those don't work, the best treatment for severe ongoing pain from lumbar stenosis may be surgery—opening of the back and side of the canal (laminectomy and partial facetectomy)—especially if leg weakness has developed.

Neurogenic and Vascular Claudication

Lumbar stenosis can cause pain and disfunction that arises from pressure on nerve roots in a tight spinal canal. Neurogenic claudication, as mentioned earlier, is a form of pain, tingling, or numbness mainly in the legs but sometimes in the back as well. It occurs while walking and is relieved by resting. Vascular claudication is leg pain that also comes from walking and stops with rest, but it does not cause back pain. This form of claudication is caused by the narrowness of arteries to the legs. When leg muscles don't get enough blood from such stenotic (narrowed) arteries during the increased demands of exercise, they cramp and are otherwise painful. Neurogenic claudication is so similar to vascular claudication that it's hard to tell them apart from the patient's history alone. To make matters worse for diagnosis and treatment, in some people both conditions exist.

Armed with a patient's history and studying the anatomy of the spine and possibly blood vessels, a doctor can identify the sources of claudication. MRI, CT, and possibly CT/mye-lograms are generally used to evaluate spinal stenosis. If the pulses in the feet and ankles, behind the knees, and in the groin are good, the arteries delivering blood to the legs are open and receiving blood from the larger arteries within the abdomen, above the legs. This suggests that the source of claudication is probably lumbar stenosis and should show up on MRI of the spine. The vascular supply to a limb can be studied using various noninvasive means. When both spinal and vascular problems are present, deciding which condition to fix first is a matter of judging the individual patient.

STENOSIS IN THE UPPER BACK AND NECK

Stenosis is most common in the lower spine, followed by the cervical spine. It is rare in the thoracic spine. Cervical stenosis is both simpler and more complicated than lumbar stenosis. It is simpler in that it is caused mainly by bulging disks that calcify. They compress the canal and foramen and also the cord and possibly the roots from the front. The facets may develop osteophytes, bony protuberances that narrow the foramen but not the canal. Unlike the lumbar spine, the ligaments in the back of the canal (ligamenta flava) are unimportant as a cause of cervical stenosis, since they are thin and bulge into the canal only insignificantly when the disk at a given segment degenerates.

The treatment of cervical stenosis, however, is more com-plicated than that of its lumbar equivalent because of the delicate spinal cord in the cervical canal. Pain in the neck and arms and weakness and sensory changes in the arms are not the only problems with cervical stenosis. Narrowing of the spinal canal in the neck—or, rarely in the thorax—compress the spinal cord, which can permanently damage it. Unless a root also is compressed, severe stenosis in these upper spinal areas may cause little pain. Compression of the spinal cord, like compression of the brain, causes no pain, but may cause initially painless neurological dysfunction, such as numbness, weakness, or abnormal gait because of tight muscles from spinal cord damage. Compression of nerve roots causes pain and possibly also neurological dysfunction.

Remember that in lumbar stenosis, the nerve roots are compressed in the canal and possibly in the foramen. In either case, this compression may cause both pain and neurological dysfunction at some point. In the cervical and thoracic regions, only root compression in the epidural space on either side of the centrally located cord and in the foramen will cause pain. Painless dysfunction can occur from cervical and thoracic stenosis that compresses the cord but not the exiting roots.

Patients with little pain or neurological dysfunction from significant cervical or thoracic stenosis need a thorough neurological examination and MRI at least annually to determine if the spinal cord is being damaged. Damaged spinal cords have a different appearance on MRIs from those that are compressed but not damaged. At the earliest sign that the spinal cord function is deteriorating or an MRI shows that damage is occurring, surgical decompression must be undertaken to preserve neurological function even if pain is not a significant problem.

Cervical stenosis doesn't cause claudication or exercise-related pain or nerve damage. This is because, among other reasons, the canal cannot become as narrowed in the neck as in the lumbar spine without damaging the cord. The cord is far more vulnerable to pressure than the roots of the cauda equina. Once the cord is significantly damaged, there will be enough arm or leg weakness to prevent exercising, so claudication-related pain won't develop.

- Cervical and thoracic spinal-canal narrowing may compress the spinal cord and cause weakness and numbness of the arms or legs depending on the spinal level. For example, stenosis in the lower cervical area, C_7-T_1, may affect only the legs.
- Bowel, bladder, and sexual dysfunction may also occur with cord compression.
- Tightness (called spasticity) may occur in the muscles controlled by nerve fibers from the cord below the level of compression. This spasticity causes an abnormal way of walking.
- Spinal cord damage is often suspected if reflexes are brisk in the knee and ankle—they jump—when the doctor taps them with a hammer.
- Pain, weakness, and numbness from root compression in the thoracic area is not easily perceived by patients or general physicians.

A recent patient had an excellent decompression and fusion of the cervical spine but still had severe signs of cord dysfunction. Her cervical spinal cord showed no signs of injury or scarring on the postoperative MRI, so the rest of her spinal cord was evaluated to try to discover another cause of her symptoms. An MRI and myelogram showed that her midthoracic cord—around the lower tip of the shoulder blades—was severely compressed by stenosis at three levels. She also needed to have these levels decompressed.

DIAGNOSING SPINAL STENOSIS

As stenosis becomes symptomatic, it often causes back or neck pain as well as radicular pain when it causes compression of nerve roots. One or both sides of the spine may be involved, and the symptoms do not always perfectly match the stenosis. Surprisingly, people with stenosis affecting the spinal canal and foramen on both sides may have only one-sided pain. This is clearly a challenge for the thoughtful surgeon contemplating how big a decompression to perform.

People usually don't get evaluated for spinal stenosis until they have pain. Then it may be found that they have not only pain but also weakness and sensory and reflex changes. Many patients have clearly had years of stenosis without severe enough symptoms to complain about until at some point they began to experience pain. Despite complaints of only three-months' duration, for example, MRI evaluation of their spine may reveal severe stenosis that required years to develop.

Plain X-rays of the lumbar spine may reveal spinal slippage, degenerative disk disease with facet-joint arthritis and foramenal narrowing, but that won't completely explain your symptoms. X-rays can't show the interior of the spine. Stenosis is a condition affecting the spinal canal and foramen.

MRI scans may be helpful in identifying nerve-root and spinal-cord impingement.

CT scan is better than MRI at showing the bony osteophytes that exist with spinal stenosis and gives better images of the small foramen in the neck.

A CT/myelogram with flexion/extension views is the best study to have before surgery. It is the only test that demonstrates the influence of bodily position on the stenosis. This is important because some areas of stenosis that appear mild to moderate when you lie straight on the myelogram table, appear moderate to severe when you bend backward. Predictably, bending forward makes the stenosis appear less severe.

A stubborn neurological colleague had three levels of stenosis and needed surgery. He felt that he needed only to be decompressed and was adamant that he didn't need a myelogram. He was operated on without it, and two levels were successfully decompressed. However, his surgery was less than optimal because the remaining level of stenosis still compressed his roots, especially when he walked. A year later, he finally had a myelogram, which revealed moderate to severe stenosis in extension, although it appeared to be only moderate when he lay flat. An operation on this last level made him significantly better, allowing him to walk without significant back or leg pain.

Patients with multilevel spinal stenosis should have myelograms before surgery.

Carefully performed diagnostic root blocks may help corroborate a clinical impression gleaned from the patient's history, examination, and radiological findings.

One test that is often not very helpful for those with stenosis is the EMG. As we age, roots at various spinal levels are irritated or damaged enough to show up on an EMG as abnormal. This may help to distinguish a root problem from one caused by peripheral nerve damage.

Regardless of test results, the correlation between symptoms and anatomic changes may not be as close in spinal stenosis as it is in most herniated disks. This has important implications for the role of surgery in the treatment of spinal stenosis.

Because stenosis can occur at multiple levels of the spine and more than one level may be causing leg pain, careful correlation between symptoms and radiographic findings is essential to determine the critical areas. In most people with symptoms of root compression from stenosis or disk herniations—or anything else—an excellent neurologist or spine surgeon should be able to identify the source of pain and dysfunction and outline various plans for treatment, including a surgical option.

TREATING SPINAL STENOSIS WITHOUT SURGERY

Treatment of spinal stenosis starts with becoming educated about the mechanics of your spine and the way your symptoms increase and decrease. You will understand why you bend over a shopping cart in the supermarket to avoid leg pain, or why your neck and arm pain feels better when your neck is bent forward. Symptoms of lumbar stenosis are reduced if you sit down, flex at the waist while walking and standing, and reduce the length of walks. But you can't sit, flex, or take only short strolls all the time. This is where drug therapy comes in, because it can help improve function.

Acetaminophen

Good old acetaminophen (Tylenol) may be as good a painkiller as the more expensive and toxic NSAIDs mentioned below. The major risk of excessive acetaminophen use is liver and kidney toxicity. However, when used in proper doses—fewer than 4,000 milligrams (mg) daily—it is safe, as you can tell from its widespread continued use. This is twelve regular strength (325 mg) or eight extra-strength (500 mg) tablets. But if you have hepatitis, don't take acetaminophen, nor if you drink a lot of alcohol, which is already hard on the poor liver; continued high doses of acetaminophen is a bad idea.

Nonsteroidal Anti-inflammatory Drugs (NSAIDs)

Nonsteroidal anti-inflammatory drugs (NSAIDs) reduce inflammation and therefore the pain it causes. Since stenosis is not an inflammatory disease, it is not clear that these drugs should be any better than acetaminophen in treating the pain from root compression, and they might be worse. The NSAIDs can cause the same type of toxicities as acetaminophen but can also erode the lining of the upper digestive tract. The major cause of death from traditional NSAIDs is gastrointestinal bleeding. Each year thousands of people die in the United States and Canada from NSAID use—not necessarily abuse. Newer NSAIDs—the COX-2 inhibitors—may be especially helpful to older patients who are at risk of developing gastrointestinal problems, but note that they, too, are not perfect. They may still cause severe side effects. (See Chapter 17 for more on these medications.)

The reality is that for significant pain from disk herniations or stenosis, most patients need narcotics or possibly short courses of oral or epidural corticosteroids to obtain relief. Unless you have medical problems that preclude anesthesia and surgery, if you require this kind of pain regimen for stenosis, consider having surgery.

Narcotics

Narcotic painkillers are the mainstay drug treatment for moderate-to-severe stenosis pain and are safer when used as directed than NSAIDs. Yet most people suffer from not getting enough of such medication because the doctor, the patient, or the patient's family fears addiction. Drugs like Percocet, Vicodin, morphine, MS Contin, Kadian, Oxycontin, and Duragesic patches are highly effective in controlling pain. For difficult-to-control pain, narcotics can be combined with NSAIDs, Tylenol, or other drugs. Read Chapter 17 for details on dependence, tolerance, and addiction and how narcotics are most effectively used.

Oral Corticosteroids

Short courses of oral steroids—about two weeks—may help someone with stenosis pain take an important trip that would be otherwise impossible. They almost always have to be combined with narcotics to achieve enough relief to make this possible. I will not give more than two such courses annually. The benefit of oral steroids may be supplemented with epidurals in patients with mild-to-moderate lumbar or mild cervical stenosis.

Steroids are inappropriate long-term therapy for treating the symptoms of stenosis. Steroids are not benign. They can cause bone loss, cataracts, ulcers; they can result in the destruction of your hip joint, diminish your ability to fight infection, produce diabetes, and increase the glucose in people already diabetic. They can cause mental disturbances and insomnia.

Unlike some diseases—such as rheumatoid arthritis—which require long-term steroid use to suppress immunity, stenosis can better be treated otherwise. If your pain from stenosis is enough for a physician to consider long-term steroid use to alleviate it, you should have surgery instead.

Epidural Injections

Lumbar epidural corticosteroid injections may help back and leg pain from mild to moderate lumbar spinal stenosis at one level. The same applies to cervical spondylosis at one level if it is mild. Attempting a cervical epidural with the large needle in a very narrow cervical segment with the spinal cord under pressure (from stenosis or a large disk herniation) is a prescription for damaging the cord and risking permanent neurological dysfunction. Cervical epidurals are more commonly used to treat pain from small cervical disk herniations. (In many cases epidurals and similar injections are performed more accurately and safely when guided by the use of fluoroscopy or a CT scanner.)

The sequence of injections is different for spinal stenosis from that for herniated disk because the underlying abnormalities are different. With a herniated disk, acute inflammation occurs as a result of toxic substances oozing out of the torn annulus and chemicals that are part of the inflammatory process that is degrading the herniated disk fragment. These chemicals irritate the spinal root, usually already damaged and swollen from pressure from the disk herniation. To wash away the toxic chemicals, quiet the inflammatory process, and reduce the swelling in the compressed roots, epidurals are given as up to three injections in a short period of time.

Stenosis is a chronic condition caused by hardened or calcified structures impinging on nerve roots. Roots compressed within a stenotic spinal canal or foramen are not inflamed but may swell from the pressure, a common response to compression by the brain, spinal cord, and roots. Unlike disk herniations, which usually improve without surgery, stenosis always goes in one direction: it always gets slowly, inexorably worse. Therefore, epidurals given for mild or mild-to-moderate stenosis must be spaced, usually given as three or four over twelve months to stretch out the effect of the treatment over the year. They do not work in moderate-to-severe stenosis, especially if it affects multiple levels of the spine. And of course it is dangerous to do epidurals in a highly stenotic cervical spine. If you also suffer from an exacerbation of pain from disk herniations, the course of epidurals may be modified as appropriate.

Susan, sixty-eight, had significant spinal stenosis at multiple levels. An orthopedic spinal surgeon had advised an operation to "open" the levels that were compressing her nerves thus causing leg pain that limited her walking. Susan did not want surgery since she was afraid it might not work. Instead, she chose to alter her lifestyle, take pain medications, and have epidural corticosteroid injections every three to four months for about two and a half years. This eased her pain so she could got to her health club for regular workouts. Limited in the standing position, she was functional seated, so she regularly rode a stationary bicycle at least four days a week. Eventually, the injections and her oral pain medication became ineffective, so she gladly accepted the risks of surgery, which was successful.

As a rule, I never advocate epidurals for stenosis patients who take blood thinners because they would be at risk for a stroke or blood clot in the lungs. However, if you are going to risk a stroke, do it for the definitive procedure, surgery.

Radiologically Guided Root Blocks with Epidurals

If you are one of the significant minority of people with multilevel stenosis who is not responding to medication and cannot have surgery for medical reasons, repeated nerve-root blocks or multilevel epidurals may help relieve pain for three to four months. They should always be performed using CT guidance because it allows the doctor to see precisely how the medication, mixed with a radiological dye, covers the multiple areas of stenosis. I use transforamenal blocks (multiple injections at various levels into the foramen around the roots and into the side of the epidural space) and epidurals as needed, so I am able to cover all the areas of stenosis at multiple levels in one session with excellent results. While labor-intensive, this technique gets dramatically better results than the typical blind epidurals performed in the office one injection at a time without X-ray guidance. Such precise and complete administration of epidural and foramenal steroids is impossible without CT guidance plus a measure of skill and determination. Such injections can be applied to the cervical or thoracic spine as well if needed. Not only may these injections ameliorate pain for several months; they may temporarily improve mild weakness or numbness. None of these injections can restore neurological function that was lost because of damaged spinal cord, however.

I have done this to various patients, at times with good results, for several years. However, this is not an acceptable treatment for a typical patient with stenosis to whom *all* of the above conditions do not apply.

Implantable Pumps for Pain Medication

In extremely rare cases—when nothing else works to relieve pain—a pump can be implanted in the back to receive pain medication. The pump is placed under the skin and connected by a small tube, also tunneled under the skin, to the lower spine. There the tube is secured in the dural sac that holds spinal fluid so that it delivers pain medication—narcotics and local anesthetics—into the fluid. The medication then works on pain receptors in the spinal cord and, possibly, the brain to block pain impulses from the lower part of the body. The pump has to be refilled once a month or so. This is not an acceptable treatment for the overwhelming majority of patients with spinal stenosis. In my opinion, if a patient can have the pump implanted surgically he can have lumbar decompression with sophisticated medical and anesthetic support.

I recently saw a woman with excruciating back and leg pain from severe lumbar stenosis. She also had severe emphysema and both diabetes and osteoporotic vertebral fractures. The latter two were caused by the corticosteroids she needed to control the emphysema. She had had a pump implanted but was still in severe pain and immobilized in bed at home—bad for her osteoporosis and her life in general. Her doctors told her she would not survive surgery. I disagreed and brought her to New York University Medical Center. With the help of colleagues, I stabilized the woman to the point that I could perform a vertebroplasty. (See Chapters 13 and 18.) We did this before surgery to strengthen the bones to be decompressed and also those above and below them. She then underwent an excellent decompression and eventually received in-patient rehabilitation. Her pain lessened, and she was tapered off from the pump. She still has a complicated spine and medical condition but went from being in pain—despite the bed rest and the intraspinal pump—to being able to walk and care for herself. She does require occasional oral narcotics for residual back pain.

WHEN SURGERY IS NECESSARY

When pain from stenosis interferes with everyday life, especially with walking or standing, or the legs or arms become weak, surgery to decompress the stenotic areas of the spine is indicated. With a skilled surgeon, results from decompression for lumbar and cervical stenosis are usually good. Greater difficulty exists when multiple levels of stenosis are present and clinical symptoms occur throughout the back and leg. However, three or four levels may be decompressed by a skilled surgeon with gratifying results.

Cervical and Thoracic Decompression

Cervical-canal stenosis is decompressed from the front of the neck and is followed by a fusion. The surgical procedure to accomplish this is refined and gives good results.

Foramenal stenosis in the neck or thoracic spine can be treated by simple operations (foramenotomies) performed from the back; they also give good results. Thoracic-canal stenosis may require decompression and fusion, often through opening the chest, a more elaborate procedure. Like the lumbar spine, multilevel stenosis in the upper spine is more complicated to treat but can be with excellent results.

Lumbar Decompression

Lumbar decompression surgery is better for the relief of leg pain caused by spinal stenosis, and it may also alleviate lower back pain if it is truly caused by stenosis, not painful facets, scoliosis, or spinal instability. Acute pain usually stops a few days to a few weeks after surgery, depending on the type of surgery performed.

Surgical procedures to alleviate pain caused by pressure on spinal roots in patients with stable lumbar spines include:

- Laminectomy removes the lamina, the bony arch in back of the vertebra, overlying the ligaments at the back of the canal.
- Laminotomy is a smaller operation that opens a portion of the lamina.
- Medial facetectomy shaves off one-third of the facet to make more room for roots compressed in the side of the canal or entrance to the foramen.
- Foramenotomy opens the foramen to relieve pressure on a nerve root.

Depending on your anatomy, part of one or both of the laminae—bony arches of the vertebrae surrounding the spinal nerves—the ligamenta flava (calcified or not) inside the spine and part of the nearby facets are drilled off. This removes the pressure on the nerves. The bones are left open, and the overlying muscle and skin is closed.

Laminotomy or laminectomy for stenosis (as opposed to disk surgery) should always include shaving off the inner part of the facets, further opening the spinal canal and foramen. Opening tight foramen that cause symptoms is important to the success of stenosis surgery. (Foramenotomy can be performed in the neck or thoracic spine with good results.) The main reason stenosis surgery may fail is the inadequate removal of the inner facets and opening of the foramen.

When Lumbar Fusion Is Necessary

People with stenosis and gross instability (spondylolisthesis) require decompression and fusion. However, patients with stenosis and stable, low-grade spondylolisthesis may be decompressed without resorting to fusion by select, skilled spinal surgeons. The majority of patients with stenosis do not require surgical fusion. Remember this: people with lumbar stenosis are the fastest-growing population subjected to surgical fusion, but the majority should not have to undergo it. Remember also that the data on outcome of lumbar stenosis surgery in this chapter is for those who don't need fusions. For those who do, fusion surgery can be beneficial, but they are likely to have some degree of long-term postoperative pain. Read more about fusion in Chapter 19.

Risks of Surgery

Decompression for stenosis carries the same risk as spinal-disk surgery: spinal-cord damage (in the cervical and thoracic spine), nerve-root damage, incontinence, bleeding, or infection. There are a few added risks for those patients who are elderly. These include an occasional postoperative lumbar or thoracic vertebral compression fracture and lumbar slippage (spondylolisthesis). Both these conditions may require further invasive treatment, including vertebroplasty and even surgical fusion.

After Surgery

It is normal to have pain after the operation. It will be most severe at the points in your spine where the surgery was done. This is caused by swelling of the previously compressed nerves as well as from the surgery itself. There may be muscle spasms across the back, neck, and into the legs or arms. Your surgeon will prescribe pain medications, including a short course of oral or intravenous corticosteroids and narcotics if needed.

If you are fit following surgery, you will be encouraged to walk right away and do gentle exercise. But avoid excessive bending, lifting, or twisting for six weeks to several months to minimize the risk of spinal slippage following surgery. If you had no slippage before surgery and the narrowed spinal segments causing pain were opened sufficiently (but not excessively), you should be well within a few weeks. If you had low-grade slippage before surgery and were not fused during the stenosis surgery, it will take several months for the spine to heal completely. Don't risk destabilizing your spine and inviting a reoperation with fusion. However, fear of possible (as opposed to probable) instability after stenosis surgery is not necessarily a reason for fusion. Stenosis surgery can usually be done without fusion with good results— and should be.

If you are out of condition from not having walked for weeks or months, it may be necessary to have some rehabilitation before you leave the hospital. A physical therapist, working under the direction of a physiatrist (a physician who specializes in physical medicine and rehabilitation) may have to help you stand, walk, and climb stairs. He or she will also instruct you in the proper way to get in and out of bed, sit and stand, and sleep.

The Results of Decompressive Surgery for Stenosis

At least 65 percent of the people who have this type of surgery for lumbar stenosis report reduction of pain and significant improvement in daily activities. When people don't do well with lumbar stenosis surgery—30 percent to 40 percent—it is often because they have an insignificant opening of the facets or foramen or have so many spinal problems that it is impossible to safely address all of them in this way. I view routine stenosis surgery as a good operation for people who need it, regardless of age, if they are medically capable of going through it. Remember that stenosis is usually a condition of aging spines, often accompanied by disk degeneration and arthritic abnormalities at multiple levels. The most severe problem, the one causing the present symptoms, may be corrected in one operation with excellent results.

In cervical stenosis surgery, at least 85 percent of patients have good to excellent results.

Thoracic foramenotomies are beneficial, and patients undergoing these procedures have little long-term postoperative pain. Thoracic stenosis surgery, if it requires fusion, may solve the problem of a compressed spinal cord—preserving or restoring neurological function—but some of these patients have significant chronic pain after it.

After several years, stenosis symptoms may recur as the degenerative process that originally produced it continues. Some people need more than one stenosis decompression in their lifetime.

Key Points about Pain from Stenosis

- Aging can lead to degeneration of the disks and facets and to calcification and bulging of ligaments inside the spinal canal, thus causing the narrowing of the canal and foramen that is known as spondylosis or stenosis.

- Spinal stenosis may cause pain, weakness, difficulty in walking, and compression of the spinal cord.

- Stenosis is most common in the lumbar spine, least common in the thoracic spine.

- About 10 percent of people are born with a narrow spinal canal (congenital stenosis) and as a result are more likely to develop back problems.

- Most people don't know they have stenosis until they have pain or other symptoms.

- The pain of lumbar stenosis can be controlled for years with medication and modification of activity.

- When stenosis pain in the back and legs is induced by walking and relieved by resting, it is called neurogenic claudication.

- A CT/myelogram with flexion/extension views is the best way to assess spinal stenosis before surgery.

- When pain or neurological damage from stenosis cannot be relieved, surgery is needed to decompress the appropriate tight areas of the spine.

Chapter 13

Osteoporosis of the Spine

One of my elderly male patients—an esteemed rabbi—survived gastric cancer only to suffer severe back pain that was insufficiently controlled by high doses of narcotic and other medication even after several weeks. His X-rays and scans showed no recurrence of cancer, but he had significant spinal arthritis, osteoporosis, and several osteoporotic compression fractures. I recommended vertebroplasty to strengthen the vertebral body that caused his most severe back pain. But we'll get to that later.

The spine, along with the hip, pelvis, and wrist, is a primary location for osteoporosis. Osteoporosis, a natural consequence of aging, is a serious public-health threat to more than 28 million Americans. When bones decalcify, the vertebrae weaken. This can result in small cracks in the vertebra to a severe vertebral crush fracture. It can also cause microfractures that produce a low-grade crunch.

Osteoporosis is more common in women. There are an estimated five hundred thousand vertebral compression fractures annually in the United States. They affect roughly 15 percent of postmenopausal women, causing pain, disability, and a reduction in height. Less than one-third of these fractures may be symptomatic. The most severe consequences of osteoporosis are hip fractures, which happen to more than three hundred thousand people sixty-five or older annually.

When osteoporosis affects the spine, the vertebrae may collapse. This leads to pain and eventually to stooped posture, a bulging abdomen, and difficulty in walking. Weakness, numbness, and other problems may also occur if spinal roots or, more rarely, the spinal cord is damaged by the collapsed bone. Treating these neurological problems often requires surgery.

Bone is made up of a framework of collagen similar to the girders of a building. Calcium and phosphorus form a mineral compound that cements the layers of the girders. Bone is continuously changing. Some cells (osteoclasts) excavate, others rebuild (osteoblasts). Our bones are the source of calcium for the bloodstream, which carries it through the body so it can play its role in a number of functions, including muscle contraction. When we are young, calcium is absorbed and stored in bone. The building cells, the osteoblasts, predominate. As we age, the excavating cells, the osteoclasts, are more active. This is how we lose calcium. If the calcium content becomes too low, the bone is weakened and is at risk for fractures. Bone also becomes less elastic and stiffer with age, further increasing the risk of fractures.

Lack of calcium in the growing years directly contributes to loss of bone mass, and many people do not get enough calcium after childhood. In adolescence they lose interest in drinking milk, and they do not replace the milk with such calcium-rich foods as yogurt and cheese or green vegetables, nor do they take supplements. Too much protein, caffeine, and phosphates from soft drinks also deplete bone minerals.

Osteoporosis is a two-stage process. Clinically significant osteoporosis is when fractures begin to occur. Preclinical osteoporosis is decreasing bone density. Here, you are on the edge of disaster, waiting for the fractures to begin. If fractures have occurred in the thoracic spine, kyphosis—dowager's hump—may be present. This is the exaggerated forward curve of the thoracic spine that pushes the head forward. (However, the most common cause of patients' assuming a bent or kyphotic posture as they age is disk degeneration.)

Risk Factors

Insufficient calcium in the diet and lack of exercise can lead to osteoporosis, but the major cause in women is untreated menopause. Other risk factors include:

- increased age
- estrogen and testosterone deficiency
- amenorrhea, or lack of menstruation (occurs in anorexic women and in some athletes)
- smoking, which robs women of natural estrogens and inhibits the action of estrogen on many organs, including bones
- history of bone fractures
- family history of osteoporosis
- white race
- low body weight
- long-term use of corticosteroids, such as prednisone, for the treatment of autoimmune conditions and chronic asthma, which can cause osteoporosis and neutralize the effect of the sex hormones, thus reducing bone density
- prolonged use of thyroid-replacement medications, some antiepileptic drugs, the intravenous blood thinner heparin, tetracyclines, and some other medications, which have similar effects to corticosteroid use

- excessive bodily production of parathyroid hormone for various reasons

Fortunately, osteoporosis caused by drugs, menstrual irregularities, or menopause can be prevented or minimized through appropriate timely medical therapy.

Symptoms and Signs

The first sign of serious osteoporosis is usually a fractured vertebra in midspine. The simplest everyday action may bring this on. A woman bends over to pick up a piece of paper from the floor. Rising from a stooped posture, she experiences sudden paralyzing back pain. She is eventually taken to a hospital. X-rays reveal washed-out bones, at least one of which is collapsed, thus explaining the pain. She is admitted and put to bed. If she is lucky, she'll be given enough narcotics round the clock to make her comfortable. If she is not analgesically blessed, she'll be given NSAIDs and some minor pain-relievers, insufficient in quantity, and will suffer terribly. Some physicians will try to put a brace on the patient, which may help a bit, or it may just make the patient uncomfortable. Within a week, the pain will usually begin to subside; the healing process may take three months.

Severe osteoporosis can also exist silently, only to be discovered accidentally. A fifty-five-year-old veterinarian friend told me he went to his doctor with a cough that wouldn't go away. Concerned about pneumonia, the doctor ordered a chest X-ray. He came back to his patient with two pieces of news. First, my friend didn't have pneumonia; he had only a nasty bronchitis. However, he did have an extraordinary case of osteoporosis, about which he was totally unaware.

Unfortunately, all the research on the treatment of this disease has been done in women, so doctors give men the same drugs women use to control their disease (except for estrogen, of course). That strategy may undergo refinement as we learn more about male osteoporosis.

Because osteoporosis is a silent disease, most people don't know they have it until they have a vertebral or hip fracture. Some vertebral fractures are seen on MRIs or X-rays of the spine taken for other purposes, such as evaluation of pain radiating down the leg when walking. Sometimes these fractures can occur silently or after a minor fall with little pain. Why some are painful and others are not is not clear. Here are some subtle symptoms:

- discovering that you are not as tall as you once were
- back pain
- stooped posture
- bulging abdomen

DIAGNOSING OSTEOPOROSIS

If you think your back pain might be from osteoporosis, or you are at risk of developing it because you take medications like cortiosteroids or because of hormonal changes, have your bone density checked.

Bone-Density Tests

Dual energy X-ray absorptiometry (DEXA or DPX, depending on the manufacturer of the equipment) distinguishes bone from soft tissue and measures the density of the spine and thigh bone. Photons that penetrate your spine or hip as you lie on a table register on a sensitive record. The computer calculates the mineral density of each bone. From that record, the doctor can tell whether your bones are above or below the fracture threshold.

Your bone density is compared with the expected density for a normal young adult and also a person of your own age, weight, and race. For example, if a forty-two-year-old woman had 91 percent of the expected peak bone density of a young woman, she is not at an increased risk of fracture. Another woman, fifty-eight, measured well below the bone density of a young woman and is therefore very susceptible to fractures.

Bone densitometry techniques are not designed to pinpoint the cause of bone loss; they measure the degree of loss. The combination of bone-density measurement and a chemical measure of bone resorption levels of cross-links in urine (see below) enable us to know if there is sufficient ongoing bone loss to cause a nontraumatic fracture, to assess risk of future fractures, and to provide a baseline for monitoring and follow-up treatment.

Cross-Link Testing

We also need biochemical markers—cross-links—to assess the rate of bone turnover and to measure effects of treatment. Urine tests for cross-links can tell us how fast we are using up bone. Cross-links, also called N-telopeptides, are breakdown products of bone. As bone turnover occurs, some of the digested bone components appear in the urine. Cross-links are more specific for bone than other chemicals that used to be measured. The test can be repeated every three months, so we can evaluate more quickly whether a treatment is working; people respond differently to different treatments.

TREATING SPINAL COMPRESSION FRACTURES WITHOUT SURGERY

Most compression fractures usually heal in two to three months, needing only pain medications during that time. Back pain after that is the result of your spinal anatomy's having been altered by the fracture. Increased pressure is placed on the facet joints attached to the fractured vertebral bodies. The facets in or even around a fracture often become chronically painful and should be treated with pain medication or radiofrequency lesions (see Chapter 18) rather than vertebroplasty (see below).

If the pain from an osteoporotic compression fracture doesn't diminish after two weeks or you decide not to control it with narcotics and other medication because of the worrisome effects, consider vertebroplasty or its related procedure, kyphoplasty, which strengthens and straightens the spine after a vertebral fracture.

This procedure is appropriate in only 10 percent or less of people with osteoporotic vertebral fractures. It is overused in the United States, sometimes by inexperienced physicians. If a few tablets of Tylenol with codeine or even much stronger narcotics daily for several weeks provides sufficient relief (with few side effects), you don't need vertebroplasty. Patients with severe pain following a compression fracture often require hospitalization and high doses of oral narcotics; they may even need intravenous narcotics for a few days to a week.

Treatment with Vertebroplasty

Vertebroplasty rebuilds bone by injecting liquefied bone cement into the collapsed bone. In a matter of minutes the liquid hardens, stabilizes the bone, and prevents further collapse. It also reduces pain. (See Chapter 18 for more on this procedure.)

Vertebroplasty may be performed on an outpatient basis or overnight in a hospital. Interventional neuroradiologists usually perform the procedure, although any physician trained and experienced in performing vertebroplasty using radiological guidance can do so.

Vertebroplasty definitely benefits the compressed vertebral body. However, in patients treated for a fracture with vertebroplasty, the risk of a new fracture in the vertebrae surrounding the treated one doubles. Remember that in an osteoporotic spine, all the vertebrae are osteoporotic, not just the one that fractured and was injected. Once the cement hardens, the injected vertebra increases the pressure on the surrounding vertebrae.

Being exceedingly conservative, the rabbi I mentioned earlier refused to have any procedure with a degree of risk, even the minimal risk of vertebroplasty. I controlled his pain as best as I could with medication. He was also on medication to prevent further bone-mineral loss but understood that that would not be helpful for several years.

The rabbi came back three months later because his pain was worse than ever. I didn't understand why he hadn't healed. Then new scans showed that one of the vertebral bodies that caused the original pain had collapsed more. Now it was pressing on a nerve root that travels under the lowest rib on the right. This resulted not only in severe back pain but also burning and aching lower abdominal pain.

The rabbi now wanted a vertebroplasty, but I knew that at this point it wouldn't work. New scans revealed that his bone was crushed in such a way that the cement would leak out into the epidural space and possibly compress his spinal cord or crush the already damaged nerve root. Also, a vertebroplasty would not take the pressure off his nerve root from the collapsed vertebral body. What the rabbi needed was sur-gery—a laminectomy and foramenotomy—to drill the bone away from the root. It worked. In a few weeks, the rabbi was back to going to daily religious services and teaching, the joy of his life. We were all thrilled. I will always wonder whether if he had had the vertebroplasty when he first saw me, he could have avoided the operation. I'll never know. Even now, I am not sure he did the wrong thing by waiting.

Treatment with Kyphoplasty

Kyphoplasty is identical to vertebroplasty except for the manner in which the cement is placed in the vertebra. It is supposed to restore the shape of the collapsed vertebra, improving not only its strength but also straightening the collapsed spine, something vertebroplasty never was intended to do and cannot do. I am unconvinced that kyphoplasty can deliver on its promise of improved spinal form, and most of my colleagues agree. Vertebroplasty therefore continues to be the preferred minimally invasive treatment for vertebral osteoporotic compression fractures.

TREATING OSTEOPOROSIS BY HALTING BONE LOSS

As you age, you need to increase your calcium consump-tion. In general, it is impossible to get all you need from diet alone. Most people are not going to drink a quart or more of milk each day or eat several pounds of broccoli. People over fifty need 1,500 mg a day. Taking calcium supplements of 500 mg three times daily is a standard regimen for increasing calcium intake.

For those at risk for osteoporosis, Vitamin D intake should be about four hundred international units (IU) a day unless you are out in the sun a lot. For those who already have osteoporosis, eight hundred IU daily should be taken. This supplementation is especially necessary in winter and in the higher latitudes. Vitamin D is needed to absorb calcium in the intestine. Without Vitamin D, calcium would be completely excreted in the stool. Many calcium supplements are available with Vitamin D added.

Too much protein can cause calcium to leach from your bones and be excreted in the urine, so reduce the amount of meat, fish, and dairy in your diet. Phosphate, such as is contained in soft drinks, also prevents calcium absorption.

If you have a predisposition to calcium-containing stones in the urinary tract, ingestion of calcium in food or supplements may compound the problem. Consult your doctor about diet and supplements. Calcium can also interfere with the absorption of other drugs and minerals, such as iron, zinc, fluoride, beta-blockers, and bisphosphonates, such as Fosamax.

Calcium Alone Is Not Enough

Osteoporosis is really a disease of adolescence that manifests itself in late adulthood. The major behavioral changes that must be introduced early are calcium intake and weight-bearing physical activity. No matter how much calcium and Vitamin D you consume, it will do you no good unless you exercise against gravity. In paralyzed patients on respirators, whatever calcium they get is excreted in the urine. Astronauts exercise significantly but not against gravity. As a result, they suffer bone resorption during their weightless missions. Likewise, swimming is good exercise but not for osteoporosis; the water helps to hold you up, thus reducing the force you must exert to overcome gravity.

The best treatment is prevention. Until recent studies showed that estrogen-replacement in women hasn't lived up to its earlier promise, indeed might be dangerous, that was the first line of treatment to prevent osteoporosis in women.

The specialists who treat osteoporosis advise which calcium supplements and medicines are the most effective for an individual. Nonprescription vitamins and minerals, such as Vitamin D and calcium, are usually not enough. All of you naturists who hate taking chemicals should realize that over-the-counter products must be supplemented by prescription medications to help restore bone density.

Available therapies include estrogens and selective estrogen receptor modulators (SERMs) for women, bisphosphonates, and salmon calcitonin for both women and men. A new agent, Forteo, is synthetic parathyroid hormone. Forteo stimulates osteoblasts and therefore bone growth. Fluorides have effects similar to Forteo's but are no longer used because of a paradoxical increased risk of fractures in 20 percent of those taking them. The other drugs mentioned above inhibit osteoclasts and therefore bone breakdown. All of these therapies carry a risk of toxicity. Discuss the choices with your physician. Don't put it off: the time to reverse the effects of osteoporosis is now.

Rheumatologists and endocrinologists are the best ones to treat this disease. Unfortunately, once a painful compression fracture occurs, strengthening the bones is the least of your concerns. You will want your pain controlled immediately. And it should be.

Bisphosphonates

Until very recently, estrogen was the only FDA-approved viable option for the majority of people susceptible to osteoporosis. Now, three similarly effective drugs, called bisphosphonates, are FDA-approved for the use in the treatment of osteoporosis. They are alendronate (Fosamax), risedronate (Actonel), and pamidronate (Aredia). The first two are administered orally, the third intravenously. They appear to be equally effective.

Bisphosphonates interfere with the function of mature osteoclasts, which break down bone. Alendronate, marketed first, is a thousand times more potent than an earlier bisphosphonate, etidronate. It increases bone density and mass while also slowing the rate of bone loss. After six days the drug becomes buried inside the bone tissue and no longer affects the osteoclasts, so it must be taken periodically.

An international clinical trial of alendronate in various dosages was carried out in almost a thousand osteoporotic women. At the end of two years, spinal bone density in those taking the drug increased by about 7 percent. It was effective regardless of age, race, and baseline bone density. Alendronate reduced incidence of vertebral fractures by 48 percent and slowed progression of vertebral deformity and loss of height.

Food impairs alendronate absorption, so you must take it at least an hour before breakfast with a full glass of water. After you take it, you must not go back to sleep or even recline, as it may cause esophageal irritation and heartburn. Since calcium and magnesium impair its absorption, calcium-rich food and supplements must be taken at a different time.

Risedronate is taken the same way. Remain upright for thirty minutes after taking it. This helps you get the full dose and reduces the risk of heartburn or damage to your esophagus. Be sure your doctor knows what else you are taking, such as vitamins or other medications. You need to get enough calcium while you take this drug, so your doctor may want to be sure your diet contains enough or may prescribe supplements.

This medication has some very rare side effects, such as

gas, bloating, constipation, diarrhea, upset stomach, leg cramps, acid reflux, bone or joint pain, or sinus infection.

Aredia is used in treatment of painful bone metastasis of breast cancer and myeloma. It's also the first drug that has been proven to reduce the formation of bone metastasis in these cancers, thereby reducing the need for chemotherapy and radiation. It's also used to treat Paget's disease.

Calcitonin is a hormone produced by special (parafollicular) cells of the thyroid gland. It tones up the calcium level in the blood and pulls it into the bone-forming area. Because salmon calcitonin is much more potent than human calcitonin, it is therefore the one used for prevention and treatment of osteoporosis. Because it is broken down by gastric acid, it cannot be taken orally. It must be given by injection or inhaled through the nose.

When given by injection, calcitonin is administered daily or three times a week. It is used in the treatment of osteoporotic fractures because it also has some pain-relieving properties. The nasal preparation is less effective than injections.

Tamoxifen is an antiestrogen that is given to breast cancer patients to inhibit the regrowth of the cancer. It has an effect on the bone like that of estrogen, though weaker. It is an alternative to estrogen for osteoporosis. Tamoxifen has side effects, however; it increases the risk of endometrial cancer and blood clots.

Evista (raloxifen hydrochloride), a newer drug that binds to estrogen receptors while not stimulating the uterus or breasts as estrogen would, may help combat osteoporosis in those who cannot or should not take estrogen. For example, raloxifen does not encourage endometrial overgrowth but does have the good estrogen effects on the bones and the cardiovascular system. Raloxifen promises to be an excellent alternative to tamoxifen. Raloxifen reduces bone breakdown and slows down the whole process of bone turnover. A thirty-six-month study of 7,705 postmenopausal osteoporotic women, aged thirty-one to eighty, showed that treatment with raloxifen increased bone-mineral density in the spine and hip and reduced the risk of vertebral fracture by 30 percent to 50 percent compared with a group treated with an inactive substance.

Forteo was approved by the FDA in December 2002. It is a synthetic form of parathyroid hormone (PTH), one found naturally in the body. It is used for about a year for severe osteoporosis to build up bone to the point where less potent agents can be used. It is suitable for men and women at high risk for osteoporosis. Forteo comes in a disposable pen device and is injected once a day into the thigh or abdominal wall. One pen contains a twenty-eight-day supply. You must be instructed in its proper use in order to assure the right dosage. In clinical trials, Forteo lowered the risk of spinal fractures and increased bone density in postmenopausal women with osteoporosis. There have been no long-term trials yet.

WEIGHT-BEARING EXERCISE

Bones need a workout to make them strong. Weight-bearing exercise—that which resists gravity—builds bone. Walking and running help build strong bones. So does walking down the stairs to give bones a good pounding. Bones that are not being used are reabsorbed by the bone-eating osteoclasts. On the other hand, when you walk you put stress on the bones of your legs, pelvis, and spine. This stress causes an electrochemical (sometimes called piezo-electric) current to bring in more calcium and bone-building materials to the area of stress. Bone-building osteoblasts go to work, and bone deposition begins. These two processes, bone formation and bone resorption, recur throughout your life. In adolescence, formation predominates over resorption. Later, at the bone peak—around age thirty—they are equal. In old age, resorption predominates, and we lose bone. The stress of bearing weight stimulates bone formation.

Vigorous aerobic weight-bearing exercise, such as walking, running, or weight lifting, for at least thirty minutes a day is the minimum recommended by the American College of Sports Medicine. Walking one to two miles daily in about half an hour helps preserve bones. When you run or walk, keep your arms loose and unencumbered by bags or packages. Walking during daylight helps you manufacture Vitamin D in your skin, essential for absorption of calcium from the gut.

Key Points about Back Pain from Osteoporosis

- The spine, along with the hip and wrist, is a primary location for osteoporosis.
- By the time you have back pain from osteoporosis, you may already have had painless vertebral compression fractures.
- A bone-density test will reveal how much bone loss you have in your spine.
- Most vertebral compression fractures heal on their own in two to three months, as you take pain medications.
- Vertebroplasty puts liquid bone cement into vertebral bodies to prevent further collapse. It is not suitable for everyone.
- You can prevent further bone loss through medication and weight-bearing exercise.

CHAPTER 14

Benign and Malignant Spinal Tumors and Cancer Pain

A high school boy who was an avid football player and wanted to become a physical fitness teacher and coach had back pain every day. Worse, it significantly impaired his sleep. Although it came on slowly and progressed, he assumed that he had pulled a muscle in his back at sports or that his bed was a problem. Nothing he did and nothing his coach told him to do helped. Aspirin dulled the pain, but it always came back. Plain X-rays of his spine showed nothing. Finally, he came to me. We did an MRI and CT scan that revealed an abnormality in the upper right sacrum, where he had the pain. A bone scan showed an osteoid osteoma, a benign bone tumor that often affects young people. After it was surgically removed, his back pain went away, two years after his pain began. That was many years ago. Today, a tumor as small as his can be burned away using a radio-frequency electrode guided by CT scan in an outpatient procedure.

Tumors that originate in the spine are rare and occur mostly in young people. Such primary tumors are usually slow-growing and benign. It is more common for spinal tumors to be metastasized from cancer in other parts of the body. That's why cancer patients should report any new complaint of back pain.

TUMORS OF THE SPINAL COLUMN

A tumor is a swelling, a collection of cells with no purpose that grow more quickly than the surrounding tissue. Benign tumors are slow growing and will not spread throughout the body. Malignant tumors can grow and spread rapidly— locally and throughout the body, destroying whatever they invade. Many tumors arise in the vertebra, both benign and malignant. They are rare but require specialized care from neurosurgeons, spinal orthopedists, neurologists, oncologists, radiotherapists, and pain-management specialists. They also require the attention of interventional neuroradiologists, who plug up the vessels in tumors with catheters passed from an artery in the groin to the tumor blood vessels. This is called embolization.

Benign tumors include osteoid osteomas, osteoblastomas, osteochrondromas, hemangiomas, aneurysmal bone cysts, and giant-cell tumors. Chordomas, affecting the area of the sacrum and coccyx in the lower spine, are benign under the microscope and rarely metastasize to other parts of the body, but for all practical purposes they are malignant. They recur and repeatedly invade the same place no matter what is done to them. True malignant tumors include sarcomas of various types arising in bone and tissues that hold the body together. These range from the slow-growing chrondrosarcoma to far more rapidly growing tumors. Some giant-cell tumors may on occasion develop into a sarcoma.

All these tumors must be evaluated with various radiological studies; occasionally a piece of them is taken with a needle to be analyzed. Later, they may be embolized—their blood vessels plugged shut—if they have a large blood supply. They may be removed surgically, which, unless they are very small, usually requires removal of the affected vertebra, resulting in destabilization of the spine, and requiring surgical fusion as part of the tumor removal. Most benign tumors are perfectly curable this way. Sarcomas are cancerous and aggressive. Spinal sarcomas are difficult to treat even with the above combined techniques plus radiation and chemotherapy.

If you have any of these unusual tumors, go to a medical center with a lot of experience in treating them.

Tumors of the Nerves and Their Coverings

Benign tumors of the coverings of the nervous system include neurofibromas, which affect the coverings of the nerve roots, and meningiomas, which affect the covering of the cord, the cauda equina, and the roots exiting the sac that contains spinal fluid. Benign tumors in the cord include ependymomas and hemangiomas. Malignant tumors in the cord include various types of gliomas and some ependymomas.

All of these tumors should be surgically treated by an experienced neurosurgical team. If it is malignant, it should be treated in a center with special expertise in this area.

Metastatic or Vertebral-Column Tumors

These tumors come from cancer elsewhere in the body. Metastatic tumors most often come from breast or lung cancer in women and prostate or lung cancer in men. They invade the vertebrae and surrounding tissue. Because these come from advanced cancer in other organs, the pain can be controlled by removing pressure on the nerve roots, preserving neurological function, and fixing any structural instability of the spine with fusion.

Diagnosing and Treating Spinal Tumors

A complete physical and neurological examination is needed to diagnose spinal tumors. Various radiological tests should be ordered. An MRI and possibly a CT scan of the suspected area of the spine is necessary. MRIs of the entire spine, one of the brain, CT scans of the chest, abdomen, and pelvis, mammograms, and bone scans may be needed to screen for other tumors in the body if cancer is suspected because of the patient's history, physical examination, other tests, and the appearance of the tumor on the available radiological studies. If a tumor is part of a newly diagnosed metastatic cancer or a cancer that has been treated in the past, the cancer will have to be staged, using the studies described above to evaluate the extent of cancer throughout the body, including bone, organ, and brain and spinal involvement. Staging is a diagnostic determination of how widespread and aggressive the cancer is so that appropriate treatment can be applied.

Sometimes a biopsy—a piece of the tumor is taken by a needle inserted with the help of X-ray guidance into the tumor through the skin—may be necessary to establish its type and whether it is from a systemic cancer not otherwise readily apparent. Biopsies may also be obtained from an open surgical procedure. The removed piece of tumor is analyzed by a pathologist with a microscope to determine its nature.

Total removal of a benign tumor is always preferred as long as vital tissues are not sacrificed. The spinal cord is highly sensitive; avoiding damage to it is a critical part of surgery. Monitoring techniques must be used throughout the surgery to evaluate the function of the spinal cord as the tumors are removed. The abnormal tissue is examined under the microscope to determine whether it is benign or malignant. Therapy depends on the diagnostic evaluation. If a tumor cannot be completely removed—if it is in the cord or adheres to many important spinal nerve roots, for example—postoperative radiation therapy may improve the outcome.

After surgery, rehabilitation can help nerves to fully heal, although it may take some time.

Malignant spinal tumors need a multidisciplinary approach. You need the expertise of a neuroradiologist, a pathologist, an interventional radiologist, a neurooncologist or oncologist, and a spinal surgeon. A pain-management specialist may also be part of the team. Some tumors that damage the spinal cord may need to be surgically removed, at least in part. This is true for some malignant tumors of the spine and some metastatic cancers that affect the spine. Treatment may also include radiation, chemotherapy, or embolization. Many malignant tumors require more than one type of treatment. Even after surgery, radiation, chemotherapy or both may be needed to further shrink them. Steroids may be needed to reduce pain and improve the function of roots and the cord that were compressed by tumors or after surgery. Pain medication, including narcotics, may be necessary to control it.

BACK PAIN FROM METASTASIZED CANCER

Cancer strikes older people more often than younger ones, and they are subject to more sources of pain. Sometimes the pain of other conditions like osteoporosis or arthritis masks or conceals the pain of a cancerous tumor that has developed. Conversely, people sometimes fear that their pain indicates cancer when the source of it is something else. When a man who has been told that his prostate cancer is in remission wakes up with terrible pain in his back, he may fear that his cancer has metastasized. However, he is just as likely to be experiencing the pain of arthritis. He should not make his own diagnosis.

Cancer cells may travel from the primary tumor through the blood vessels or lymph channels to other sites of the body and form new, secondary tumors or metastases. These tumors may destroy bones, possibly resulting in painful fractures. They may compress or damage nerves, causing severe pain, weakness, numbness, and possible bladder and bowel dysfunction. Much of the pain from cancer is a sign that a tumor is damaging something.

Diagnosis

Any new pain without a known cause that persists for several weeks deserves examination by an experienced physician using high-quality diagnostic MRIs or CT scans, supplemented by other tests as needed, such as plain X-rays and bone scans. If you have a history of cancer, any new pain should be considered a possible recurrence of the cancer until proved otherwise.

- Blood tests, such as the prostate specific antigen (PSA), may indicate the presence of a tumor. Similar tests monitor breast and ovarian cancer.
- Plain X-rays of a painful area may not identify the tumor unless there is significant destruction of bone.
- A bone scan is sensitive but nonspecific for identifying the cause of bone lesions: benign tumors, malignant tumors, arthritis, fractures, and infections.
- An MRI is the most sensitive for finding metastases

in the vertebrae, spinal cord, roots, and surrounding muscles and organs.
- Whether a biopsy of the tumor is done depends on various clinical and radiological factors.

In order to treat pain most effectively, an oncologist and often a pain specialist experienced in treating cancer patients must diagnose the type of pain, such as burning, throbbing, or aching, and the source or sources of it. It may be from damaged muscles, ligaments, tendons or bones, or nerves, feeding internal organs. Therapy must be directed at controlling pain and treating the cancer.

TREATING BACK PAIN FROM METASTASIZED CANCER

Today in 75 percent to 80 percent of cancer patients, pain can be adequately controlled by narcotics or other pain relievers given orally, rectally, or in skin patches. For the few who need more pain relief, intravenous or subcutaneous narcotics may help. On average, only 10 percent or less of cancer patients require extraordinary, high-tech means of pain control, such as injecting narcotics into the spinal canal or, when all else fails, destroying the nerves that carry the pain impulses from the body to the spinal cord or brain.

Pain from new or progressive cancer must be treated not just with pain medication but also with anticancer agents directed against the malignant tumor that is causing the pain. Conceptually, this is no different from giving painkillers to reduce pain while preparing a patient for getting a broken bone set or for surgery to remove a large disk herniation that is causing sciatic pain and disability. Pain treatment must occur in conjunction with treatment of the disease. This is why patients with cancer pain are treated most effectively with a multidisciplinary approach that includes adequate analgesic drug therapy, anticancer therapy, neurosurgical and anesthetic pain-relieving procedures, behavioral methods, and supportive care. Interventional treatments may occasionally include lesioning nerves or nerve roots, and rarely the spinal cord or brain; plugging up tumor blood vessels; and vertebroplasty.

Treatment with Radiation

Radiation therapy is frequently highly effective in quickly and efficiently treating cancer pain from tumors of bone, internal organs, and nerves, and it has few side effects. Improved radiological devices (MRIs, high-quality CT scans) make it easier to see exactly where tumors are and better techniques of focusing and delivering radiation. Radiation therapy aimed at a painful tumor-ridden bone relieves pain in 70 percent to 80 percent of patients in a few weeks. Patients with pain from bone metastases from breast, lung, and prostate cancer make up about 20 percent of referrals to radiation therapy departments. Therapy can be given in a shorter or longer course, depending on the patient's tumor type and condition. Theoretically, a high dose single course of radiation can relieve pain in twenty-four hours and has no more long-term side effects than a longer course.

Another form of radiation helpful in treating bone pain from metastatic cancer, particularly from prostate and some breast cancer tumors, is in the form of radioactive isotopes. In the past strontium[89] was used but was phased out in favor of the more effective samarium[153]. Injected intravenously, it is incorporated into areas of osteoblastic or malignant activity in bones. It impairs the growth of certain tumors in bones and relieves pain. However, this form of therapy takes three to four weeks to work and may damage the marrow where blood cells are made. This limits severely the ability to tolerate any future chemotherapy, which also often attacks the marrow. Therefore, these isotopes are usually given as a last resort.

Treatment with Chemotherapy

Even when chemotherapy doesn't cure cancer, it can prolong life and control tumor-related pain by shrinking tumors. Most chemotherapy has side effects, such as nausea and hair loss, which are not painful and can be controlled with medication or which subside with time. Some may damage peripheral nerves outside the spine and result in pain or weakness.

One patient who had lymphoma ten years ago continues to suffer from numb, painful feet. He therefore takes narcotics and a tricyclic—an antidepressant that treats the pain from damaged nerves—with excellent results, but he takes them constantly. However, he never doubts that the trade-off—lifesaving chemotherapy for the lymphoma for numb painful feet later—was worth it. Chemotherapy saved his life, and the aftereffects are well controlled by the medication. He is a prosperous plumber in New York with a loving wife and two fine children. Not such a bad outcome, is it?

Treatment with Corticosteroids

Corticosteroids are used to shrink certain kinds of cancerous tumors, such as lymphoma. They can shrink swollen nerves and a spinal cord compressed by tumors, just as steroids do when these structures are compressed by disks or narrowing of the spine. The spinal cord, nerve roots, and peripheral nerves become swollen under pressure, producing pain and loss of feeling or other nerve damage. By shrinking nervous system structures that are under pressure, pain or numbness is reduced. Steroids also significantly reduce pain from bones damaged by tumors.

Steroids also combat the negative effects of nerve tissue (spinal cord, nerve roots, peripheral nerves) that swells during or following cancer treatment. (As it dies, the tumor swells temporarily.) This side effect of successful anticancer therapy may further compress surrounding nervous tissue, temporarily worsening pain and neurological function.

Steroids may be given in a short course or, if the tumor cannot be eradicated, may be given for months. Unfortunately, they weaken the muscles and bones and may cause diabetes among other complications. Also, the body becomes habituated to them after long use; when they are withdrawn, they can cause other problems.

Treatment with Narcotics

It has been shown that 90 percent of cancer patients can get adequate pain relief from the skilled use of various kinds of painkillers, including narcotics, given through noninvasive or minimally invasive low-tech means. Yet a 1993 study of oncologists revealed that 76 percent of those surveyed felt that they insufficiently evaluated pain complaints. Only half believed they were able to control patients' pain in a good or very good fashion. A majority admitted that they were hesitant to prescribe enough narcotics to control their patient's pain. The undertreatment of cancer pain may be diminishing, but it is still a problem, as is the inadequate treatment of all moderately severe pain.

Even in selecting the best medication to reduce pain, the source of the pain should be considered. Pain from tumor invasion or distortion of internal organs is treated with narcotics as a mainstay of therapy (other medications may be combined with the narcotics as needed). Adding other drugs to the regimen allows good relief with less use of narcotics. For muscle and bone pain, narcotics should be combined with medications such as NSAIDs or Tylenol. NSAIDs reduce inflammation and NSAIDs and Tylenol pain from tumor invasion. Corticosteroids also reduce inflammation and swelling (see above).

Bone pain from tumors can also be relieved significantly by adding corticosteroids to a narcotic regimen. For pain from compression of tumors on the nerves, corticosteroids, tricyclic antidepressants, and antiseizure drugs in conjunction with narcotics—when necessary—are remarkably helpful.

Medication usually has to be given in progressively more invasive ways as the disease progresses. Giving narcotics under the skin (subcutaneously), intravenously, or into the spine are three means of providing increased pain relief. For a given narcotic, the more drug that reaches the spinal cord quickly, the greater and quicker the pain relief. A drug arriving at the brain is more likely to result in side effects, such as sleepiness, nausea, vomiting, and a diminished ability to breathe. Here, briefly, are some ways narcotics can be delivered to relieve cancer pain. (For more in-depth information, see Chapter 17 on the delivery of narcotics.)

Skin patches. One of the advantages of the Duragesic skin patch is that the narcotic in it—fentanyl—is delivered through the skin into the fat under the skin and eventually into its tiny blood vessels, from which it goes to the central nervous system. Because it bypasses the digestive system, it does not produce constipation, a common side effect of narcotics. After the patch has been used for a day, it works smoothly, providing a constant dose of narcotic without the wait of forty-five minutes that pills require before they begin working. Even when patches are changed, pain relief continues fairly smoothly because there is still a reservoir of narcotic stored in the fat under the skin. (This is different from using oral medication. Once the effect of the pill begins to wear off, it takes forty-five minutes for a new pill to begin working, creating more of a see-saw effect.)

Subcutaneous and intravenous routes, while invasive, are even more efficient. Narcotics introduced directly into the bloodstream are three to six times more potent than oral drugs. Intravenous narcotics begin working within minutes. Very high doses of narcotic may be given in a constant infusion this way. This technique is important in treating severe pain, especially if it has suddenly occurred, as with a malignant tumor that results in a fracture of the spine. External pumps are used to deliver narcotics through these routes. Patients are increasingly familiar with the use of patient-controlled analgesia (PCA) devices after surgery. They deliver a fixed amount of narcotic per hour and offer the option to the patient of injecting extra narcotic every ten to fifteen minutes, say, for flare-ups of pain not controlled by the normal infusion. This system is also used for delivering narcotics through various invasive (intravenous, epidural) routes to cancer patients.

Intrathecal and epidural infusions of narcotic, occasionally combined with local anesthetics, are delivered to the spinal fluid (intrathecal) or the fat around the dura (epidural). These infusions are carried out through catheters tunneled under the skin and muscle; their tips wind up in the spinal fluid or the epidural space. They may be attached to a temporary external or long-term indwelling pump, which delivers the medication at a controlled, adjustable rate. External pumps may offer PCA as well. When they are put directly in the spinal fluid that bathes the cord, they are a hundred times more effective than the same dose given intravenously. Delivering it to the epidural space—the fatty area around the spinal cord—is ten times more effective than by the intravenous route. In either case, less narcotic is needed for the same pain-relieving effect and results in fewer systemic side effects. (Systemic means throughout the body.)

Treatment with Drugs that Prevent Bone Breakdown

Both bone pain and excess calcium in the blood from bone breakdown caused by cancer's spreading to them can be helped with any of a class of drugs that prevents bone breakdown. (One such as Aredia.) Some of these drugs are used to fight osteoporosis. Aredia is particularly useful in treating bone pain, excess blood calcium resulting from breast cancer, and a blood cancer called myeloma.

Treatment with Other Drugs

Nerve-related, or neuropathic, pain, which is more common than bone pain in cancer, is less responsive than bone pain to narcotics used alone. When necessary, medications for nerve pain should be integrated into a multidrug pain-relieving regimen. This can minimize this difficult-to-treat, all-too-frequent type of cancer pain. Aside from the corticosteroids mentioned, nerve pain may be treated with anti-seizure medication, some antidepressants, and some heart drugs. Oncologists often overlook the best drugs for neuropathic pain.

Vertebroplasty and Other Interventions

Vertebroplasty is an excellent way to relieve cancer-caused bone pain in a small percentage of well-selected patients before, during, and after antitumor therapy. It is a technique for strengthening fractured or collapsed vertebral bones with a quick-drying liquid cement. This makes the bone stronger and prevents further collapse, and it relieves pain. The technique is used to treat painful vertebral collapse from cancer, osteoporosis, or hemangiomas in the vertebrae. It can also be used for hips affected by metastatic cancer.

Over 75 percent of patients treated with vertebroplasty for cancer experience significant and rapid reduction of pain and improved ability to function in a day and can live on less pain medication. (See Chapter 18 for more about this procedure.)

I still vividly remember the first patient I treated with this technique after returning from France where I learned it in 1993. Beth Samuels, fifty-two, was referred to me by an oncologist for control of pain from cervical cancer that had spread to her lumbar spine. Beth had significant low-back pain that radiated into her right leg. Her pain was only modestly controlled by a regimen of several drugs that included high doses of narcotics. Her cancer had slowly advanced over the past two years until incapacitating back pain made it impossible for her to sit through a movie, one of her pleasures. She had maximal radiation therapy to the painful spine and had been on different forms of chemotherapy for the previous two years. The oncologists had exhausted the available chemotherapeutic regimens, and her cancer continued to advance. Beth knew she was going to die of her disease but at least wanted to improve the quality of her life for the time she had left. When she did not have significant low-back pain, it was because she was sedated from narcotics.

Four of her lumbar vertebral bodies had metastatic cancer, and I felt that most of her pain originated in those bones. After extensive radiological studies, I decided it was feasible to place bone cement into the affected bones, using special needles pushed and hammered into place under CT guidance. I told her I preferred this technique to the ineffective pain treatment—intraspinal narcotic therapy—because vertebroplasty might not only relieve her pain; it might strengthen her tumor-ridden bones, preventing them from collapsing further. (An ongoing collapse would eventually give her more pain.) An added benefit of this technique in patients like Beth is that it may slow the growth of tumors where it is injected. Beth was willing to try anything. It was a good thing that she did try it. The vertebroplasty worked; within two days she was able to sit through *Gone With the Wind*. Yes, better living with vertebroplasty, but remember that it is appropriate only for some patients. Most sent to me for this procedure are totally unsuited for the treatment.

Fewer than 5 percent of patients may require other therapies: destroying nerves damaged by tumors caused by toxic chemicals like alcohol and phenol; radiofrequency lesions of ganglia (the sensory computers of nerves near the spine) damaged by tumors; or lesions of the pain pathways of the spinal cord or brain itself; and angiographic embolization (plugging up blood vessels) of tumors affecting the spine. Lesioning nerves or pain pathways cuts off the barrage of pain signals from damaged nerves to the brain. Embolizing tumors in and around the spine partially cuts off their blood supply, causing them to shrink and thereby reducing damage to bones or nerves affected by them. All of these procedures carry the risk of creating additional damage to the nervous system and more pain, weakness, and numbness than previously existed.

WHEN BACK PAIN IS CAUSED BY CANCER TREATMENT

In one study, slightly over a quarter of patients had pain from cancer therapy: surgery, chemotherapy, and radiation. Every time you have an operation, nerves are pulled, pushed, and cut, usually with no long-term ill effect. Some body areas are more likely to cause significant postoperative pain, occasionally permanent. This kind of pain is usually a result of nerve damage or scarring. Some are more likely to experience such scar formation than others. Extensive neck surgery for control of cancer may lead to a constant burning pain in an area of diminished sensation on the outside of the neck. Removal of a kidney can cause back, abdominal, and groin pain if the lumbar nerve is damaged. All postoperative pain requires medication or other treatments to control it.

Radiation damages nervous tissue and causes problems in fewer than 5 percent of patients. I recently saw as a patient a fellow physician. He had developed throat cancer, which was cured by surgery and radiation. However, the radiation damaged his spinal cord behind his throat, leaving him with disabling pain from his neck down.

Chemotherapy if properly given usually does not damage the spine and usually has no effect on the cord or roots. It may affect peripheral nerves, as already mentioned.

It is imperative to diagnose pain resulting from cancer treatment and distinguish it from pain from recurrent or new malignant tumor growth.

Key Points about Spinal Tumors and Cancer Pain

- Benign tumors can cause back pain.
- In cancer patients, most back pain comes from cancer that has metastasized from other organs.
- Most cancer pain is underreported and undertreated.
- More than 60 percent of cancer pain is caused by a tumor invading tissue.
- At least 75 percent of cancer patients can get relief from back pain with some combination of narcotics and other pain medication.

Chapter 15

Recognizing and Treating
Other Causes of Back Pain

Many medical conditions unrelated to the spine can cause back pain. Problems in nearby organs in the genito-urinary and gastrointestinal systems can cause referred back pain. Anyone who has had a kidney stone is familiar with severe colicky pain characterized by repeated spasms of intense pain followed by periods without any. This kind of pain comes from spasm in hollow structures, such as the ureter, colon, or gall bladder. Kidney and gall bladder pain occur in the upper portion of the lumbar spine; colonic pain occurs lower down, near the sacrum.

Pregnancy and menses cause varying degrees of temporary back pain in women. Inflammatory diseases affect the spine, ankylosing spondylitis being the most conspicuous example. Rheumatoid arthritis causes pain and even serious neurological dysfunction in the uppermost spine. The pain of fibromyalgia may occur in the back, too, and also the limbs.

The important message here is that back pain should never be treated without a diagnosis. Is it from spinal arthritis? Or is it referred from an undiagnosed malignant abdominal tumor or a lung tumor that has invaded the thoracic spine?

It can often be difficult to determine the causes of the different types of back pain. The job is made more difficult because the same person can experience pain from more than one cause.

FIBROMYALGIA

Fibromyalgia (FM) can be confused with other causes of back pain, especially facet-related pain—with which, indeed, it may coexist—and simple muscle pain. Fibromyalgia is a soft-tissue pain syndrome characterized by chronic pain in discrete tender point areas, including the lumbar spine. Widespread chronic pain lasts at least three months. It includes muscle pain and tenderness, with several points that are especially tender to the touch spread over both sides of the body, above and below the waist. These points may be on the limbs and also the neck, thoracic area, or lower back. These tender points are not the trigger points seen in typical myofascial pain, and the tender areas of fibromyalgia have a more symmetrical and widespread distribution than myofascial pain, which usually occurs in only one side of the body in a discrete area. Fibromyalgia may also cause tension headaches, irritable bowel syndrome, and low blood pressure on standing up after lying down or sitting.

Still poorly understood, fibromyalgia is recognized more readily than in the past. About 80 percent of people with this disease are women. Although it initially occurs at age twenty to sixty, juvenile onset accounts for 15 percent to 25 percent of the cases. The pain of FM may be unremitting, with durations of up to twenty years; or the discomfort may wax and wane. Reasons for this variability are unclear.

The onset of FM often seems to follow an injury, excessive physical activity, or another painful condition. In one study 22 percent of patients who suffered a whiplash injury in an accident developed FM within a year as compared with 1 percent of those who sustained leg fractures. It may be that the length of time pain exists has something to do with the development of FM: The pain from a broken leg usually goes away in six weeks, but whiplash pain may persist for years. Supporting this hypothesis is that some chronically painful conditions may make some patients more likely to develop fibromyalgia. For example, some data indicate that 20 percent to 35 percent of people with rheumatoid arthritis or lupus (also inflammatory conditions) also suffer from fibromyalgia. It is also commonly seen in people with chronic low-back pain or common wear-and-tear arthritis.

Some chronically painful conditions may sensitize the central nervous system (brain and spinal cord) and trigger or maintain an abnormal response to otherwise painless sensations. Once the nervous system is sensitized, all sorts of normally painless stimuli can hurt. Therefore, it is not surprising that patients with fibromyalgia also have a greater likelihood of suffering from other painful disorders that have no apparent cause: female urethral syndrome, irritable bowel syndrome, and restless leg syndrome.

However, if 20 percent to 35 percent of people with some chronic inflammatory conditions and similar percentages of those suffering from chronic whiplash pain develop fibromyalgia, why do the majority of those with these conditions not develop it? There is more to the cause of fibromyalgia than sensitization from chronic pain. Possibly there is a genetic predisposition to fibromyalgia. Maybe it is caused by exposure to some environmental conditions or other. The influences may coexist: a genetic predisposition and an environmental trigger at a crucial time in life. Fibromyalgia is common in female relatives of people with fibromyalgia.

Whether this is because of genetics, common environmental exposure, or both is not clear.

Symptoms of Fibromyalgia

Fatigue, depression, insomnia, migraine headaches, irritable bowel, and morning stiffness may all coexist with the pain. It is not clear if fibromyalgia is one disease or a collection of overlapping painful conditions. Fatigue is a prominent feature of FM; patients often report restless sleep and morning exhaustion. Cold or humid weather, overactivity, total inactivity, stress, menses, and poor sleep exacerbate FM. Symptoms generally improve with moderate activity, in warm and dry weather, and with massage.

Diagnosing Fibromyalgia

As with myofascial pain, no abnormalities that can be detected by laboratory tests reveal its presence; it is another test-negative chronic painful condition.

Areas that are tender to touch are referred to as tender points and are localized, most commonly on the upper border of the shoulders, elbows, knees, and the lumbar spine. There is no pain outside the area. There may be eighteen or more sensitive areas in someone with primary FM. Other than identifying these tender points, a physical examination usually is normal. The diagnosis of FM is made by ruling out other conditions.

The American College of Rheumatology in 1990 reported classification criteria for FM that include a history of widespread pain in four body quadrants for a minimum of three months and pain in twelve of eighteen tender points when manually palpated. In addition, the presence of another disorder does not exclude a diagnosis of FM. In a study of patients who'd had spinal surgery and were referred to a spine center for lumbar pain, 12 percent had FM complicating their condition; it had not been diagnosed.

Treating Fibromyalgia

Treatment of FM requires a multifaceted approach that includes muscle relaxants, low doses of tricyclic antidepressants, sleeping pills and sedatives, and nonsteroidal anti-inflammatory drugs (NSAIDs). Narcotics should be tried for moderate-to-severe chronic pain that doesn't respond to other medications.

- Educate yourself about the illness. It can be reassuring to know that your symptoms are not all in your head. Once you know the condition is not life-threatening, deforming, or degenerating, you can adjust your lifestyle.
- Rest and relaxation are especially important if you are overworked. Keep working but avoid excessive fatigue.
- Range-of-motion and stretching exercises improve muscle function. An aerobic exercise program is essential.
- Heat treatments are also useful.
- Additionally, massage, stretching, biofeedback, relaxation exercises, and stress-reducing ergonomic furniture may all help fibromyalgia. Support groups may be beneficial as well.
- Antidepressants, such as the tricyclic Pamelor or Norpramin, which treat depression can, in lower doses, treat pain. They may also induce sleep at night without causing daytime drowsiness. Selective serotonin reuptake inhibitors like Prozac or Zoloft may help some people, but in general, this class of

antidepressants does not work as effectively in FM as the tricyclic drugs.

- Muscle relaxants, such as Flexeril, may also be helpful.

Obviously, some people with fibromyalgia may also have coexisting painful problems, such as stenosis, facet syndrome, or areas of typical, well-localized, myofascial pain with well-localized trigger points. In these cases, treatment of the coexisting painful conditions by any reasonable means is appropriate and likely to help reduce overall pain.

INFLAMMATORY DISEASES OF THE SPINE

Spondylitis (spon-dee-LYTIS) is an inflammation of the joints or arthritis of the spine. The facet joints, the disk spaces, joints connecting the ribs to the spine, and sacroiliac joints are affected. Because spondylitis is a manifestation of systemic diseases that are capable of causing inflammatory arthritis in various joints, the hip, shoulder, and peripheral joints may also be affected.

According to the Spondylitis Association of America, as many as a million people in the United States have ankylosing spondylitis (AS) or one of its related diseases: psoriatic arthritis and inflammatory bowel disease spondylitis. A significant percentage of patients with psoriatic arthritis (related to the skin disease) and inflammatory bowel disease (ulcerative colitis, and, to a lesser extent, Crohn's disease) also have spondylitis. There is no known cure for any of them, but they can be managed to be less painful.

Because they are similar and cause inflammation of the joints of the spine, these conditions are collectively referred to as spondyloarthropathies, literally, diseases of the joints of the spine.

Pain and inflammation may affect only the sacroiliac joints

or may extend through the entire length of the spine to the neck and may cause bilateral pain. Over time, chronic spinal inflammation can lead to complete cementing (fusion) of the spinal vertebrae, a process called ankylosis, which can eventually immobilize the spine. Once fused, the spine is very brittle and subject to breakage from trauma. The lower neck is the most common spot for fractures. Chronic disease can cause forward curvature of the thoracic spine and limit breathing capacity. It eventually can cause scarring of the lungs and therefore coughing and shortness of breath, especially after exercise.

AS affects all age groups, even children. The most common onset of symptoms is in the second and third decades of life. It is two to three times more common in men than in women. In women, the joints away from the spine are more frequently affected than in men.

Genetic Roots of AS

A gene called HLA-B27 occurs in 90 percent of those with AS. However, just because you have this gene does not mean you will have spinal arthritis. Other factors are involved. Though 7 percent of the Caucasian population in the United States has the gene, only 1 percent actually gets the disease. On the other hand, in Northern Scandinavia (Lapland), 24 percent of the population has the gene, but only 1.8 percent of the population has AS. Even among people with the gene, the risk of getting AS appears to be further related to heredity. In HLA-B27–positive people who have relatives with the disease, their risk of developing AS is 12 percent, six times greater than for those whose relatives do not have AS.

Variations on AS

There are several other conditions similar to AS in the category of spondyloarthropathies.

Spondyloarthropathy. Inflammatory arthritis of the spine (spondylitis) causes the proteins and white cells that fight infection in the bloodstream to attack spinal structures. The lining (synovium) of certain spinal and nearby joints swells and impedes motion. The body responds to ongoing inflammation by depositing calcium in the inflamed joints and ligaments. Erosion of bone (vertebra) around the disk joints and destruction of the disk occurs, followed by scar and bone formation. The result is a spine with fused facet joints and calcified ligaments. This spinal arthritis causes stiffness in all directions of spinal motion and tenderness over inflamed portions of the spine. X-rays of the lower spine help to identify early changes from the arthritis. This includes loss of the lumbar curve (lordosis), erosion in the sacroiliac joints, and squaring of vertebral bodies (the front of the normal vertebral body has an indentation running from the top to bottom; when inflammation erodes the top and bottom of the curve, the vertebral body becomes a square).

Psoriatic arthritis. The percentage of people with psoriasis, a common skin disease, who also develop arthritis is higher than in the general population. Spondylitis occurs in 20 percent of them, and they have varying degrees of peripheral joint pain. They usually have fewer symptoms of spondylitis than those with ankylosing spondylitis, but it can still result in severe arthritic fusion of the sacroiliac joints and spine. Most had skin lesions either before the arthritis appeared or they appeared at the same time; a small number have characteristic arthritis symptoms with no evidence of skin abnormalities. Arthritis may be present for ten to twenty years before the psoriatic skin lesions appear.

Inflammatory bowel disease (ulcerative colitis and Crohn's disease) and arthritis. Twenty percent of patients with ulcerative colitis develop arthritis. This affects the peripheral joints in 75 percent of them and causes spondylitis in 25 percent. In Crohn's disease, 5 percent of patients suffer from peripheral arthritis and/or spondylitis. The spondylitis in these patients with inflammatory bowel disease is similar to that of AS. Unlike AS, which more often affects men, the spondylitis of inflammatory bowel disease affects both sexes equally. The peripheral arthritis of inflammatory bowel disease correlates with the activity of the bowel disease. The worse the bowels, the worse the arthritis. The spinal arthritis in these patients is not related to bowel disease activity, however.

Similar Conditions

Rheumatoid arthritis is a systemic inflammatory disease that affects the upper spine, particularly the neck, after it has already attacked the joints in the hands, feet, and hips. A crippling, long-term autoimmune disease, it is generally treated with anti-inflammatory drugs and physical and occupational therapy. In more severe cases drugs are used to reduce the body's ability to destroy its joints by turning its immune system against itself.

Diagnosing Inflammatory Diseases of the Spine

With early diagnosis and treatment, pain and stiffness from inflammatory diseases of the spine can be controlled and fusing may be reduced. Plain X-rays identify the skeletal abnormalities of spondylitis. A blood test identifies genetic factors that predispose people to develop spondyloarthropathy. That you have the HLA-B27 marker associated with these illnesses doesn't mean you will get it. In women, AS is usually mild and therefore difficult to diagnose.

Treating Inflammatory Diseases of the Spine

Treatment for inflammatory diseases of the spine may include exercise, medication, posture management, self-help aids, and surgery.

- Nonsteroidal anti-inflammatory drugs (NSAIDs) reduce pain, stiffness, and inflammation and facilitate motion. They do not cure the disease.
- Oral or injected corticosteroids are powerful anti-inflammatory agents used to control spondylitis, but they can have serious long-term side effects. When the disease is unresponsive to steroids, medications that suppress body immunity are considered.
- Posture correction and deep-breathing exercises aid lung expansion. Stretching improves spinal mobility. Swimming is the preferred exercise for inflammatory spine disease because it is the least stressful on bones and joints.
- Acute inflammatory arthritis improves with the control of inflammatory bowel disease, but spondylitis does not, even if the colon is removed.
- In psoriatic arthritis, it is not clear that control of the skin disease influences its arthritic manifestations.

Spinal surgery is rarely indicated in the treatment of any of these diseases. Occasionally, patients with rheumatoid arthritis need surgery to decompress the uppermost cervical cord (at C_{1-2}), it having been compressed by inflammation in the joints connecting these vertebrae. This area also may become unstable in these patients and require stabilization by surgical fusion. Patients with spondylitis may require stabilization and fusion surgery if their (brittle) spine breaks. Because of the fragility and stiffness of these patients' spines, this is often a difficult proposition.

AS and each of the spondyloarthropathies are areas of continuing research.

Sacroiliac Joint Pain

The sacroiliac joint connects the bones of the back of the pelvis. It may be a source of pain in the sacral and buttock areas and even refer down the leg along the sciatic nerve. Common causes of sacroiliac joint pain include stepping into a hole with one leg in and one out or a direct blow to the side and back of the pelvis. Spondylitis (see above) and infection can also be medical causes of sacroiliac joint pain. Pain entities that may coexist with sacroiliac joint pain include one-sided facet pain (see Chapter 7), myofascial pain, and bursitis of the hip. You can easily tell your physician that it's your sacroiliac joint that hurts just by pointing to it. This is a reliable diagnostic sign.

Radiological studies, such as plain X-rays, CT scans, and MRIs, may reveal fractures and the medical conditions mentioned above. Aside from these conditions, there are no reliable tests to distinguish a painful joint from a painless one.

Many patients over the age of thirty have some arthritic degeneration of the joint that is not necessarily painful. Because most sacroiliac joint pain is test-negative, it is diagnosed by history and clinical examination alone.

Some physicians inject the joint capsule with local anesthetic and long-acting steroids to confirm their suspicion that it is generating pain. Injecting it may reproduce a patient's pain, only to have it relieved shortly thereafter by the local anesthetic. Long-acting steroids are also included in the injection, with the idea of relieving pain that is presumably due to inflammation of the joint over several months. I use the radiofrequency technique to lesion nerves that innervate the back of the joint with good results.

In most of my patients with painful sacroiliac joints, pain also emanates from one-sided facet syndrome, buttock myofascial pain, and bursitis of the bursa overlying the hip on the painful side. These all need to be treated, with injections, lesions, and physical therapy, depending on the pain generator, to provide long-term relief to the patient.

COCCYDYNIA

The coccyx (tailbone) is a small bony structure at the base of the spine. It is joined to another bony structure, the sacrum, by a disk of cartilage (it is a remnant of the tail that early humans had). Three small bones fused together make up the coccyx. Coccydynia, or painful coccyx, can be triggered by childbirth or by a repetitive activity, such as cycling. Coccydynia is usually caused by trauma, such as falling backward on the ice, landing on your buttocks and hitting the coccyx at the same time. The pain may go away in a few days but sometimes persists and becomes chronic. It is then difficult to treat and is often test-negative. On an MRI, some people show evidence of a healed small fracture years after a fall.

A condition called secondary coccydynia is also common. This is pain at the juncture of the lower back and the sacrum. It is a form of referred pain and should go away once the pain generator in the lower lumbar spine is treated successfully.

A painful coccyx interferes with sitting, obviously, and may therefore be disabling. Sitting on a soft surface like a pillow helps. Medication may also bring relief. Usually required is a regimen of narcotics and possibly other types of pain-killers.

Treating Coccydynia

Nerve blocks and epidurals are usually ineffective in the long run against coccydynia. Freezing the nerves of the coccyx may help for several months. Partially destroying the ganglia of the nerves to the coccyx may sometimes be useful, but there is a small risk of causing anal sphincter dysfunction. Surgically removing the coccyx almost never does anything except create new pain, possibly superimposed on the previous pain.

Several years ago, I was in Moscow at the Burdenko Neurological Institute. The doctors there asked my opinion about an unfortunate woman who had developed intractable coccydynia in a fall. As she lived six hours from the city, I never actually saw her. They explained to me that she had been treated with medication, injections, and radiofrequency lesions and finally had had her coccyx surgically removed. In spite of more medication and injections, her pain had persisted for years after the surgery. I reasoned that either she never had coccydynia at all or that somehow the pain from it had become centralized, that is, it became permanently "memorized" by or "programmed" into her central nervous system, in the pain-processing areas of the spinal cord and brain. I have no reason to doubt that originally she had pain in her coccygeal area, but I will never know whether it emanated from her coccyx, from surrounding structures, or was referred from higher up the spine. The point is that, as is usual, surgery did not help.

Is there any good news about coccydynia? In my experience, many cases of so-called chronic coccydynia from trauma are not primarily from pain emanating from the coccyx. The ligaments and muscles surrounding the coccyx are involved in the pain. Deep injections of local anesthetic and corticosteroids into these structures and muscle massage often relieve the pain for months, even years. This treatment can be repeated from time to time if needed.

INFECTION

If back pain is accompanied by persistent fever or chills, an infection may be the cause. The pain caused by an infection may progress slowly, but it can become severe. It is present even while you rest and is exacerbated by movement. Bacterial infections in and around the spine can affect the skin or muscles (cellulitis), bone (osteomyelitis), disk (diskitis), or facet joint (septic arthritis).

The source of the bacteria may be an infection in the skin or muscle remote from the spine. The bacteria travels from the initial site of infection to the spinal area, or a local wound that penetrates the flesh over the spine. One to 2 percent of people who undergo spinal surgery develop an infection at the surgical site. Diabetics, people on corticosteroids or other immunosuppressive drugs, some cancer patients, persons without spleens, and AIDS patients are especially vulnerable to infection because of immune deficiencies brought about by these conditions or their treatments.

Diagnosing and Treating Infection

Visual inspection of a skin or surgical wound should suggest infection, but that diagnosis needs to be backed up with radiological tests and by analysis of cultures from blood samples or the wound itself. MRIs, CT scans, and sometimes plain X-rays can also show the effects of presumed infection on various tissues. Bone scans can suggest infection of bone, and gallium scans can actually demonstrate that infection exists, as evidenced by white blood cells collecting in various bodily structures.

To treat infection with the appropriate antibiotic, the bacteria—far more rarely fungus—causing the problem must be identified. (Viruses do not cause the kind of infections we are concerned with here.) This can be done by growing a culture from a blood sample, probing the wound, or extracting fluid from in and around the infection with a needle.

Once the bacterium is identified, the infection can be treated with specific antibiotics.

VASCULAR ABNORMALITIES

An aneurysm of the abdominal aorta may cause a throbbing pain in the lumbar spine. The aorta is the principal arterial blood vessel that supplies blood from the heart to the rest of the body. It runs just in front of the lumbar spine. An aneurysm is a weakening in the wall of the vessel, similar to a weakening in the bulging side wall of a tire. If the pressure becomes too great, the tire may blow out; similarly, if the pressure on the wall of the vessel occurs, an aneurysm will leak and eventually rupture, at times precipitously.

There may be no symptoms with a slowly growing aneurysm, but it may be noted on X-rays of the abdomen taken for other reasons. Pain frequently increases as the aneurysm grows. People who have high cholesterol levels, are long-term heavy smokers, have high blood pressure, or a family history of aneurysm are at high risk for aneurysms.

Physical examination of the abdomen reveals a pulsating mass. X-rays will reveal the aneurysm if there is calcification in the vessel wall, and a CT scan is very good at identifying the extent and size of the lesions. Injecting intravenous dye to better determine the blood flow in the arteries around the aneurysm is a procedure that may be performed before surgery. Aneurysms of five centimeters or smaller can be watched; those of six centimeters or more require bypass surgery. This elective procedure has a 2 percent mortality rate. Mortality rises to 30 percent if the vessel has leaked. (In most cases a true rupture is fatal: You lose too much blood too quickly to survive.)

Here are some other vascular abnormalities that can cause back pain and dysfunction of the lower extremities including bowel and bladder problems.

- Arteriovenous malformations (AVMs) are a network of arteries and dilated veins that cause symptoms by shunting blood away from the normal supply to the spinal cord, usually the thoracic area.
- Vertebral body hemangiomas may cause pain and dysfunction at any spinal level. (Hemangiomas are the port wine stain you see on some people's faces.) Most don't cause symptoms unless they bulge out from the body and compress the spinal cord or a root. They are usually found incidentally on an MRI for disk herniations and the like.

AVMs and hemangiomas are treated with embolization—plugging them up—or open surgery as needed.

SCOLIOSIS

Scoliosis is a curvature of the spine into an S shape. The spine may also twist like a corkscrew (rotatory scoliosis) as it curves. Minor curvatures of the spine are common and usually don't lead to pain or dysfunction, but more severe ones often do. The cause is usually unknown. Scoliosis is most often found in teenaged girls. Some schools sponsor screening programs that identify at-risk teenagers at an early stage of curvature. Adults, primarily women, may develop the condition at ages twenty to forty. Most curvatures are stable and do not progress with age. In older people, spinal curvature may develop when disk space narrows and spinal joints degenerate.

There are several signs that suggest that scoliosis is developing:

- one shoulder higher than another
- an uneven hemline
- prominence of one shoulder blade over the other

When scoliosis is detected very early, exercise and a brace may help to avoid surgery later in life, although this is not an established fact.

When younger people develop severe curvature (more than forty degrees), slow spontaneous progression of the deformity results. Progressive curvature has consequences: Vital organs in the chest and abdomen may be squeezed. The imbalance in the spine may also cause one leg to be shorter than the other. However, we don't know yet what degree of difference in leg length is linked to low-back pain. A heel lift under the short leg may be beneficial.

Treating Scoliosis

Noncritical curvatures are treated with exercise and medications. Young people with severe scoliosis require a thoracolumbar fusion: the placement of metal rods that stabilize the spine and reduce the curvature. This operation carries with it the risk of damaging the spinal cord resulting in permanent neurological dysfunction. This should be done only by experienced scoliosis surgeons, who usually work with a team of anesthesiologists who monitor spinal-cord function during the surgery and treat the postoperative pain. Often two operations are performed, separated by a week or so:

one in the back and another from the chest and abdomen.

Long-term postoperative pain management and rehabilitation is also important. It takes months to recover from such a surgical procedure. At times it must be repeated, with the stabilization being extended up and down the spine.

Lillian complained of increasing low-back pain after sitting for long periods at her computer. Now forty-five, she had scoliosis as a teenager. Because bracing had not worked and the spinal curve was severe, Harrington rods were placed in her spine. She had given birth to two children without difficulty, but her work now required long stints at the computer. She was concerned that the curve was getting more pronounced. When I examined her, I found that her curve was no worse than it was when the rods were inserted. However, the rods themselves can place more pressure on the ligaments, disks, and joints of the spine above and below the fusion. She had developed arthritis at these sites, so range-of-motion exercises were needed, as were daily nonsteroidal medication and occasional mild narcotics for episodes of increased back pain when she traveled. She also joined an aqua-aerobics (water exercise) program and swims three times a week. This combination therapy allows her to live normally and work at her computer with minimal discomfort.

Lillian's story should dispel the misconception that scoliosis surgery results in limited motion and a limited life. In fact, most scoliosis patients can lead normal lives, including having children, as long as their problem is identified in a timely manner.

Older patients with scoliosis may also have to undergo surgery, usually in conjunction with the decompression of stenosis or after a vertebral compression fracture. These patients fare less well than their younger counterparts. They often have significant chronic postoperative pain.

PREGNANCY AND MENSTRUATION

Half of pregnant women develop moderate-to-severe back pain. This pain can be from hormonal changes that alter the flexibility of ligaments and joints in the pelvis or simply the mechanical problem of the added weight there. The pressure on the supporting structures in the pelvis or a marked increase in the lumbar curve (lordosis), strains the supporting muscles.

There is normally almost no motion in the joints of the pelvis, the front of the pelvis, and the sacroiliac joints. During pregnancy, however, a hormone, relaxin, is produced. It allows increased motion of the pelvic joints, which causes tension in the relaxed capsule and ligaments. Increased lordosis, or forward curvature of the lower spine, also increases the stress on the muscles near the spine. Active movement, such as climbing stairs, increases the strain.

Relieving Pain

Being physically fit before pregnancy may cut your risk of developing back pain. If a pregnancy is in your future, a physical fitness program with aerobic and strengthening exercises is helpful. If you are already pregnant and have back pain, exercises and external supports can be helpful.

Here are some ways to reduce pain.

- Lie on your side.
- Exercise in a swimming pool to strengthen your muscles while limiting strain on the lower extremities.
- While standing, place your hands on the low back and bend backward.
- Lean on a table and bend backward.
- Kneel on the floor while resting your upper body on a chair and increase the curve in your back.

- If you have pain on one side of your back, lie down on the side with the pain, putting a small pillow at your waist.
- Support your abdomen by placing your hands under it and lifting gently. If your back pain is reduced thereby, you are a candidate for a corset with a flexible band in front that expands as you enlarge through your pregnancy.

Acetaminophen (Tylenol) is the only safe pain medication during pregnancy. In rare cases, a new mother may require bracing after delivery.

Endometriosis

Back pain that coincides with a woman's menstrual cycle may be from endometriosis, a disease in which tissue from the lining of the uterus (endometrium) is present outside the uterine cavity. The endometrial tissue may be on the ovaries or at the bottom of the pelvis near the rectum. Pain results because endometrial tissue outside the uterus undergoes the same monthly cycle of growth, shedding, and bleeding as the tissue inside the uterus. When endometriosis is near the colon and ureter, back pain is usually present. Pain increases at the start of menstruation and persists throughout the bleeding.

Endometriosis is often diagnosed through laparoscopy, a simple surgical procedure that allows us to view the inside of the abdomen. Internal organs can be biopsied to determine the presence of endometrial tissue located outside the uterus.

It is usually treated with oral contraceptives or other medications that suppress menstruation and thereby suppress the growth of the endometrium.

Back Pain in Heavy-Breasted Women

Women can develop back pain when the weight of their breasts forces their back to curve forward. Think of carrying a heavy backpack on your chest. You would frequently have to straighten up and pull your shoulders back to ease the strain. Breast-reduction surgery may relieve the problem, but women should consider other possibilities first. For example, wear a supportive bra with wide support bands. Try back-strengthening exercises so that your back will be better able to support the weight.

If these steps don't ease the problem, breast-reduction surgery may be the best solution. Understand that you will have scars for about two years and that your medical insurance may not pay for it: It is considered cosmetic surgery. Try your best to convince your insurer that the surgery is necessary to ease your back problems.

Key Points about Other Causes of Back Pain

- Fibromyalgia can be confused with other causes of back pain, especially facet pain and simple muscle pain, with which it may coexist.
- Anklylosing spondylitis and its related diseases cause inflammation of the spine and pain.
- Pain at the base of the spine in the coccyx can be triggered by an injury or childbirth.
- If back pain is accompanied by persistent fever or chills, an infection may be the cause.
- An aneurysm of the abdominal aorta may cause pain in the lumbar spine.
- Scoliosis is a curvature of the spine that can be painful.
- Half of pregnant women develop moderate-to-severe back pain.

Part III

Types of Treatment for Back Pain

Chapter 16

Physical Therapy and Exercise

Physical and occupational therapy can do many wonderful things in the right setting. It may help someone who is stiff or out of shape from a long bout of chronic back pain during recuperation from a car accident or osteoporotic spinal fractures. It can also help loosen a stiff shoulder after a prolonged bout of neck and arm pain from a cervical disk herniation. It can recondition people who have lost the ability to walk because of a severe accident, stroke, or amputation. Unfortunately, physical therapy is sometimes used inappropriately and unsuccessfully as a substitute for surgery.

If you have severe lumbar stenosis—a narrowing of the spinal canal that causes painful pressure on the nerves—physical therapy is not a good use of your resources or time. Similarly, one of the most absurd but common misuses of physical therapy is when one is in pain from a disk herniation. Does it make sense to rub a delicate, swollen nerve back and forth over a disk herniation the consistency of hard rubber? Not if you hope to get better. You may improve in spite of this legalized torture but not because of it. Physical therapy should be done *after* the pain from the herniation has been considerably reduced and only if you need any therapy at all at that point.

Remember that physical therapy doesn't heal anything. It does allow you to recondition yourself if you need to as you heal on your own.

USING PHYSICAL THERAPY EFFECTIVELY

As we age, spinal disks become more like pancakes than cushions, facet joints become arthritic and may limit movement, and our muscles get out of shape. We must consider new ways to use our back muscles and body position to protect our spine. A general exercise program and, where necessary, focused exercises and physical therapy can help us reach that goal.

Physical therapy must often be accompanied by appropriate pain medications so that you are able to participate fully in your rehabilitation. Although it may cause pain during and after, physical therapy usually won't hurt you in the long run. Some people feel better in the physical therapist's office, but when they go home the pain comes back. If physical therapy has not given you significant periods of relief after six weeks of treatment, you may be wasting your time and money.

After scoliosis surgery or a car accident in which you sustained multiple injuries, months of therapy may be needed, but even then you should see some gradual, continued benefit to continue it as prescribed.

Physical therapy is useful for back pain if it is prescribed at the appropriate time. If you begin too early, you are too hot, meaning that the pain is so acute that any attempt to improve movement will only increase muscle spasm and pain. Trying to stretch back muscles or doing strength exercises in the early stages of an episode of acute low back pain, for example, can cause greater pain. The time for exercises is after your pain has receded and you can move with more comfort.

Here are some reasons for completing a course of physical therapy and exercise:

- Stretch and strengthen your muscles;
- Reduce stress to your spinal structures;
- Reduce the pain from unconditioned muscles and joints;
- Improve your posture and mobility;
- Improve fitness to reduce the risk of recurrence.

Physical therapy is not magic. It's guided exercise. It mostly depends on you. (We're assuming the guide knows what he or she is doing.)

One precaution: Never confuse the role of a personal trainer with that of a physical therapist. Personal trainers have no medical training. They are simply drill sergeants, educated to varying degrees in physical fitness, who guide you to maximize your exercise regimen to improve your strength and stamina. One man at a health club complained of a sharp pain in his back during his session on a stair climber. The trainer urged him to "keep going and work through the pain." That man had a disk herniation that severely compressed a nerve. For obvious reasons, he could not work through the pain. He should have been encouraged to stop and be medically evaluated if he did not improve within a reasonable period. A physical therapist is trained to work with people who are unable to carry out daily activities because of physical pain or injury. Experienced and conscientious physical therapists are more likely than trainers to recognize disk herniations and the like that may occur during physical activity.

See a Physiatrist First

The type of physical treatment that is best for you usually should be determined by a physiatrist, a physician specially trained in physical medicine. They are the physicians most qualified to issue instructions to physical therapists. (Some spinal surgeons and neurologists may be able to write appropriate orders, but most cannot.) They may make decisions about your treatment in conjunction with other physicians who are caring for your spinal problem. Without expert guidance, you may get the wrong type of exercise with therapy and make matters worse.

Not all physiatrists—doctors who prescribe the therapy—and physical therapists are the same. Moreover, physical therapists often disregard the instructions of the physiatrist—the physician ordering the program—opting for their own idea about therapy. Being pragmatic, I really don't have any objection to the physical therapist's taking over if his treatment approach works. However, when the therapy doesn't appear to be working—and you are really doing it—you must rethink your options after several weeks of giving it the old college try. Consult with the physiatrist again and describe the therapy as you are experiencing it. If the physiatrist is disappointed with the lack of results and the therapist did not follow his direction, changing therapists is an obvious option. If you still have no luck, consider another physiatrist, or consider that the diagnosis that sent you to physical therapy was incorrect.

STRETCHING AND STRENGTHENING YOUR BACK MUSCLES

Some of your back muscles are among the biggest in your body, but they are not the strongest. You need to know how to strengthen and relax them so that they reliably give you the support you need.

No single set of exercise works for all causes of acute and chronic back pain. Flexion and extension exercises have been shown to be helpful for chronic low back pain when properly prescribed. Flexion is bending your spine forward; extension is bending it backward. Before you begin any of these exercises, check with your doctor to be sure they are appropriate for you.

Flexion Exercises

Back and leg or arm pain can occur when nerves are compressed by a narrowed foramen in a spinal vertebra. (Remember that the foramen is the hole or window through which the nerve exits the vertebra.) When you bend forward, the opening expands for the nerves, reducing the compression. This also decompresses painful facets in the back of the spine. Lumbar flexion stretches tight muscles that move the hip and low back in a backward direction and strengthens abdominal muscles that pull your spine forward. In the neck, flexion stretches the neck muscles that hold your head straight and vertical and strengthens the muscles that pull your head down and to the side.

Flexion exercises can be done on an exercise table or a mat on the floor. They must be done in a proper sequence from a resting state to stretching, then to stretching and strengthening. So it is best to learn them from a physical therapist.

- Do flexion exercises if you have low back pain that is worse with prolonged standing or sitting or if low back or neck pain is worse when you bend backward, better when you bend forward.
- Do not use flexion exercises if you have a herniated cervical or lumbar disk or have leg pain in a seated

position; they may push the disk further against the already compressed root.

Some flexion exercises are easy to do frequently throughout the day. For example, every hour or so, flatten your lower back against a wall with your knees bent. Notice how it automatically tightens your abdominal muscles. Hold this position for a few seconds. This movement, called a pelvic tilt, is also one of the best ways to stretch the muscles on the back of the spine and strengthen the front ones. You can also do this exercise when sitting, standing, or lying flat.

The Valsalva maneuver is an isometric back flexion exercise. With your mouth and nostrils closed, forcibly exhale. This action pushes down on your abdominal muscles as if you were forcing a bowel movement. Another is to squeeze the cheeks of your buttocks (the gluteus muscles) together. For a sustained pelvic tilt, do a Valsalva maneuver and cheek squeeze together. These motions can strengthen the flexor muscles and give you greater stability.

Flexing the head on the neck while seated on a stool or a chair with a low backrest in the shower can be helpful. (The hot water will loosen the muscles.) You must be seated because you won't relax your neck muscles sufficiently while standing. Bending your head forward, helped by pulling gently with the arms, is a good exercise. It should be repeated at various angles in the forward position, from right to left or vice versa, thus covering the actions of the various neck extensors. Flexing the head on the neck—bringing it forward while lying down or against resistance, such as against a cushioned wall while standing or sitting, is a good way to strengthen the neck flexors.

Extension Exercises

In doing these exercises, you are essentially bending backward. Extension exercises strengthen the muscles along the back of the spine and improve spinal mobility. This helps reduce your risk of reinjury.

Extend your low back by lying on your stomach and propping your upper body up on your elbows. Some people can't initially tolerate this position, so begin slowly. For a more advanced extension, press down with your hands while your pelvis remains on the floor. You can do this standing, too, by arching slowly backward with your hands on your hips. However, this is not as effective as is the prone position. Extending the neck gently while lying facedown or sitting or standing against a cushioned wall is a good way of strengthening the neck extensors.

- Do extension exercises if you have pain in your low back from prolonged sitting or bending forward or pain in the groin when you get up from a chair or stand. Extension exercises should follow a progression in the early phase and should be directed by a physical therapist.
- Do not do extensions if you have a disk herniation—they are liable to worsen that condition and force more disks out of place. They are also likely to make the pain of stenosis worse: They reduce the diameter of the spinal canal by forcing more ligamenta flava along the back of the canal to bulge into it.

Neck Exercises

Bending your neck sideways may be required for several cervical problems, including myofascial pain in the shoulders and arms from one group of muscles. Tension headaches from myofascial pain of the big muscle that bends the head forward and turns the neck to the side is another problem treated in part with these exercises. In them, you firmly but gently bring your ear to the shoulder, first one side, then the other. This is done while you lie down on your back with one arm behind you: Pull the shoulder down by anchoring the hand of that arm to the opposite buttock, then gently pull the head to the opposite side with the other arm. Repeat several times in each direction.

Stabilization Exercises

Stabilization exercise has become a popular method for the physical treatment of spinal pain. The focus is the control and protection of the affected area of the spine. This is accomplished by a progressive program of stationary and movement exercises. These should enable the patient to establish a safe or neutral position of the spine. This position is intended to protect the spine through guided muscle activity.

Effective Use of Exercise

The key to effective exercise is to make the muscles more efficient without damaging their cells. When you damage the cells, the muscles take longer periods of time to heal. This defeats your purpose. Finding the appropriate amount of stress your muscles need without damaging them can be difficult.

If you follow your exercise routine regularly, you are most likely to feel better and suffer less from spinal pain. Many people are able to stop their medicines and remain functional even though the beneficial response is at times delayed. For example, a forty-five-year-old carpenter developed back pain after standing in an extended posture for several hours installing a set of heavy cabinets. Thereafter, whenever he extended his spine, he developed severe muscle spasm and increased pain. He was given an NSAID and a muscle relaxant for relief of his symptoms. More important, he was educated about the need for flexion exercises and the danger of bending backward. Within a month, he was back at work building and installing cabinets, but when he stopped his medications, his back pain returned. Undaunted, he continued his exercises; after a year he no longer needed the muscle relaxant, and a few months later he stopped taking the NSAIDs. He is still working—and still doing his exercises.

TENS (TRANSCUTANEOUS ELECTRICAL NERVE STIMULATION)

Physical therapists sometimes use transcutaneous electrical nerve stimulation, or TENS, as part of a rehabilitation program and a way to reduce pain. Electrical impulses are applied to the skin through small EKG-like electrodes. While it is not a cure for pain, it may relieve symptoms in some patients. Some studies suggest that it may relieve up to half the pain in more than half the patients. It seems to work for the relief of various types of acute and chronic pain, including musculoskeletal, nerve, postoperative, and cancer pain. However, according to one high-quality study, it has no benefit in the treatment of low back pain. It's worth trying for back pain as long as you can do so in a ten-day trial at home with no financial risk. Trying it before physical therapy sessions two or three times a week does not constitute a true trial.

How It Works

The TENS impulses are delivered by a battery-powered device, smaller than a pack of cards, that you can attach to your belt. Thin wires run from the unit to electrodes placed on your skin around the painful areas of your body or on areas lying within the same pathway of the spinal nerve root that controls the painful area. The placement of the electrodes is determined both by knowledge of the pathways through which pain signals reach the spinal cord from the periphery and by trial and error.

You can activate the TENS unit at will. In one frequently used method of TENS stimulation, the unit is activated for about fifteen minutes every hour and repeated as needed. The unit can also be kept on nearly continuously, with breaks as short as three minutes between stimulations. TENS gives mild tingling or strong pins-and-needles sensations; high settings may produce muscle contractions. By increasing the intensity and length of the impulses, the stimulation spreads and deepens. Optimal response guides the most efficient setting. I try out the unit with interested patients in the office, and record stimulation settings that they find most beneficial. They then go home and experiment with the settings we discovered together.

TENS reduces pain by using one kind of stimulation to reduce the processing of pain impulses. It has an effect on pain similar to that obtained by biting, licking, or rubbing a burned finger or one squeezed by a car door. The relieving stimulation activates nerves that compete with and inhibit the processing of incoming pain impulses at the level of the spinal cord. TENS also increases endorphins, our own naturally occurring narcotics, thus inhibiting pain impulses from rising to the brain from the spinal cord. Some studies indicate that it may also affect the autonomic nervous system, which controls automatic, unconscious processes necessary for survival, such as heart rate and blood pressure and flow.

Using It Effectively

TENS is not a cure, but it may reduce painful symptoms and give you a sense of control over your pain and treatment. TENS is best used in conjunction with other therapy, such as medication, physical therapy, acupuncture, or psychological therapy. Many of my patients have used TENS with some benefit, but few have been satisfied with it over extended periods. Nevertheless, those that purchased a TENS device usually feel it was worthwhile.

No adverse effects of TENS have been documented. However, as a precaution, TENS should not be used if you have a pacemaker. It is not meant to be worn over the carotid arteries, near the eyes, or over the front of the chest (especially if you have heart problems).

Patients are frequently given TENS treatments during physical therapy sessions, thus getting a few hours of pain relief, but they are not given a unit for home use. Such a policy makes little sense for the patient who may come in for therapy only two or three times a week.

The unit most of my patients use costs about $685. Many insurance companies reimburse at least part of the price, and Medicare covers about half. Some insurers, however, regard this technique as an experimental procedure and will therefore not pay for it.

TENS does not work for everyone. People with psychological problems accompanying back pain may add to their discomfort with TENS.

AEROBICS FOR ENDURANCE AND STAMINA

As the pain from your back begins to subside, aerobic exercise will build up your endurance. If you do them regularly, you will notice that you feel more comfortable for increasing amounts of time. Aerobics most helpful for back pain are walking, swimming, and riding a stationary bicycle. Before your back pain began, you may have been running instead of walking, swimming timed laps instead of paddling in the pool, or riding a regular bicycle. Choose an exercise program that you will continue over an extended period of time.

Key Points about Physical Therapy and Exercise

- Physical therapy is the use of exercise and physical treatment methods to relieve pain and restore function.
- Do not continue any physical therapy if it makes you worse or fails to make you progressively better.
- Have your spinal physical therapy program designed by a physiatrist, or, in some cases, an appropriately knowledgeable spine surgeon or neurologist.
- Take pain medication to help accomplish the goals of physical therapy if needed, as long as the therapy is helping.
- Flexion, extension, and stabilization exercises can help stretch and strengthen back muscles and prevent future problems.

Chapter 17

The Challenge of Finding the Drug—or Drugs—That Will Ease Your Back Pain

Drugs do kill pain, but not all drugs work the same way on all people. That's why it's often hard to find drugs that work for you. Medication is useful only if physicians prescribe it appropriately and patients take it when needed. In the last century, particularly in the last fifty years, there has been a proliferation of highly effective, safe, well-tolerated pain-relieving medication. Yet despite this pharmacological advance, medication—narcotic and nonnarcotic alike—is still all too often underprescribed by physicians and underutilized by patients.

Most doctors are reluctant to treat severe chronic back pain (or any pain) with narcotics for fear of government regulations on prescribing them and an exaggerated fear of addiction fed by high-profile cases in the media (see below). These fears are even worse for those suffering from pain not from cancer. Yet narcotics are the most effective medication for the treatment of most moderate-to-severe back pain and are some of the safest pain-relieving medications when taken appropriately. Their effectiveness may be greatly enhanced when combined with other pain medication, such as acetaminophen (Tylenol).

Some painkillers work by reducing the pain impulses to which—unconsciously or consciously—your body reacts. It is as though a car alarm continues to sound even after we have closed the window and therefore cannot hear it or at least not as well. Medications that kill pain often are designed to mimic (narcotics) or manipulate (tricyclic antidepressants) chemicals in our body's pain-regulating system.

Aching pain from muscular problems or a disk herniation is treated with anti-inflammatory drugs; if severe, corticosteroids and narcotics. For a pinched nerve, narcotics, some antidepressants, and other drugs bring pain relief by inhibiting the function of specific pain-processing cells in the brain and spinal cord. These classes of drugs limit the number of pain messages that these cells can process, so you perceive less pain. The effect is similar to wearing earplugs in a noisy room. The more narcotics used, the less pain that is experienced and reacted to. For example, a surgeon can inflict excruciating damage to your body in an operation, but since you are under anesthesia, the pain messages delivered to the spinal cord or processed by the brain are significantly reduced.

When we seek to manage back pain through medication, we must determine, sometimes through trial and error, the right drug or drugs and the correct dosage for the patient. We need to take into account his or her age and lifestyle; even sometimes figure out the best time and means of administering. This process is an art, and there is more to it than we can cover here. This is why it is so important if you have chronic back pain to find a doctor who has successfully treated many patients who had difficult-to-control pain.

NONSTEROIDAL ANTI-INFLAMMATORY DRUGS (NSAIDS)

Inflammation, as seen on the skin, brings swelling, heat, redness, and pain. It comes from chemicals released from various inflammatory cells in the body that dilate blood vessels and cause them to leak a straw-colored liquid, the same liquid that oozes from a skinned knee. This causes swelling, heat, and redness. Other inflammation-related body chemicals, such as prostaglandins, irritate nerve roots in the spinal canal or nerve endings in joints, thus causing pain. Some of these cells and the chemicals they produce can destroy joints and other bodily structures. Inflammation is not always a prominent feature of spinal pain. Muscles sore from overwork or misuse, the most common cause of back pain, are not inflamed. Much facet pain may not be inflammatory, although some diseases do cause inflammatory facet arthritis (see Chapter 15). Disk herniations and annular tears, though, may cause inflammation of the nearby nerve roots.

Nonsteroidal anti-inflammatory drugs (NSAIDs) may reduce pain and whatever inflammation exists in facets and around irritated or pinched nerve roots. So the right dosage of the given NSAID may be effective in treating some spinal arthritic pain, discogenic pain, and mild pain from a compressed nerve root. Many are sold over the counter. The most common NSAID is aspirin. In addition to aspirin, NSAIDs available without a prescription include ibuprofen (Advil, Nuprin, Motrin IB) and naproxen (Aleve).

Do not confuse aspirin with Tylenol, which is *not* an NSAID. And keep in mind that Tylenol controls pain as well as NSAIDs do without the risk of stomach upset or ulcers. However, it has no anti-inflammatory properties. For many simple painful spinal conditions, Tylenol should be used as the first-line drug to control pain.

These drugs are the most widely used pain relievers. Many of them, like the ones mentioned, may be bought without a prescription. Yet they account for thousands of deaths each year in the United States and Canada in the population of arthritis patients taking NSAIDs, primarily from gastrointestinal bleeding.

HOW TO USE NSAIDS EFFECTIVELY

If one NSAID does not work, try another. Always read the label on the box to determine the safe and most effective dose. If you have taken an NSAID for two weeks without benefiting, you need to see your doctor. If you take them constantly, ask your doctor about taking higher doses of the over-the-counter ones or getting a prescription for a possibly more effective NSAIDs. Also available only by prescription are the new COX-2 inhibitors, which are no more effective than NSAIDs but have fewer gastrointestinal side effects. (Fewer does not mean none.)

At any dose, all NSAIDs interfere with the ability of the blood to clot. That's why you must stop them ten days before surgery or invasive procedures to restore your normal blood-clotting mechanism. At high doses or with prolonged use, especially in women over sixty-five, NSAIDs can cause nausea, indigestion, and ulcers. They can also cause liver and kidney damage, elevate blood pressure, and cause mild water retention—enough to put some patients with frail hearts into heart failure, a serious condition in which water accumulates in the lungs and legs.

Other Drugs for Spinal Arthritic Pain

Many people with muculoskeletal pain are undertreated: Acetaminophen (Tylenol) just doesn't do the job, or they cannot tolerate NSAIDs. Two other remedies are available for mild pain. Less effective painkillers than NSAIDs, they don't have the serious side effects.

Glucosamine, a new and totally different type of substance from the above drugs, definitely helps reduce mild pain for a while in many patients with arthritis and other musculoskeletal pain until the disease progresses and pain from it worsens. It is made from a substance taken from the shells of crab, lobster, and shrimp. It is reputed to enhance growth of cartilage and is nontoxic, but there is no evidence of its benefit in the long run. It has not proved helpful for people with severe arthritis.

Chondroitin, not regulated by the FDA, is believed to make the cartilage tough. Cattle windpipes are the source of chondroitin used in supplements. (It used to be made from shark cartilage but could be contaminated with heavy metals, such as mercury.) Now, however, there is concern about mad cow disease. There are fewer studies on chondroitin than for glucosamine; whether there is any benefit to chondroitin over glucosamine remains to be determined.

It might make more sense to use stronger and, probably, safer pain-relieving drugs, like appropriately prescribed narcotics, to control most moderate-to-severe pain in patients.

CORTICOSTEROIDS

Corticosteroids are man-made drugs that are chemically similar to active hormones produced by the adrenal glands. Because they reduce inflammation and swelling, they control musculoskeletal pain from joints, pain from pinched nerves, and pain from bones with cancerous metastasized tumors. They are far more powerful than NSAIDs. So are their side effects.

In spinal-pain control, corticosteroids are used for only a brief period of a few weeks, because they stress the stomach and because of the nature of their long-term side effects (see below). They are sometimes used for longer periods to treat some kinds of arthritis, cancer-related bone or nerve pain, and pain and nerve damage or compression from brain or spinal cord tumors.

How to Use Corticosteroids

These steroids are taken orally or by local injection to concentrate medication in one area for a while, as in epidural injections (see the next chapter). Eventually the injected medicine diffuses into the body and the local effect dissipates.

Steroid treatment reduces swelling of nerve tissue from compression by herniated disks or tumors pressing nerve roots or the cord. It also reduces inflammation that may occur around a herniation or in some cases of facet arthritis. The benefit of steroids usually begins within a day of starting treatment. They are usually given in a course of one to two weeks for pain unrelated to tumor, such as disk herniations causing nerve root compression. The positive effects of these medications may continue for several weeks. In nerve root pain from disk herniation, for example, as long as the steroids are active, pain, weakness, or numbness is dramatically reduced. The herniated disk often shrinks, and the whole situation resolves nicely. However, for an ongoing process like some forms of inflammatory spinal arthritis or stenosis, the pain eventually returns.

Side Effects

Side effects from taking oral corticosteroids for a few days or weeks or more initially may include insomnia, mood swings, gastric irritation or symptoms of reflux, increased appetite, and menstrual irregularities. Diabetics will see their glucose rise occasionally; nondiabetics may see the same result. Most people do fine on this medication for a one- to two-week course, taking antacids to reduce the gastrointestinal side effects and sleeping pills for the insomnia. In those getting injections with high-dose steroids, the most common side effects are elevation of blood sugar in diabetics and menstrual irregularities in women.

If you take steroids for more than a few weeks, the side effects are more serious and get worse over time. They include weight gain, acne, and water retention with swelling of the legs. As time passes, there is a risk of infections because of diminished immunity. A change in the distribution of fat occurs: a lump on the back of the lower neck may arise. Osteoporosis, weakness of the muscles (particularly the thighs), breakdown of the skin, and a special fracture of the hip, called avascular necrosis, may occur. (The last requires a joint replacement.) Obviously, these effects have a serious effect on the body, so the less time you spend on corticosteroids the better.

ANTIDEPRESSANTS

Two types of antidepressant are sometimes effectively used to control back pain caused by damaged nerves.

Tricyclics

Tricyclic antidepressants were originally used only to treat depression. They were later found to work on several chemical pathways of the central nervous system, where they reduced the flow of pain messages to the brain. They increase the level of two naturally occurring substances—serotonin and norepinephrine—in the brain and spinal cord. These substances inhibit the neurons in the spinal cord that transmit pain signals up to the brain so it processes fewer pain impulses.

Pain can be treated with a far lower dose of these tricyclics than is prescribed for psychiatric reasons. Also, the pain-relieving effects become apparent within five days (the antidepressant effect, at higher doses, may not begin for several weeks). It therefore appears that they work differently and on different parts of the central nervous system in alleviating pain rather than depression.

For spinal pain, the tricyclics—such as amitriptyline (Elavil), nortriptyline (Pamelor), and desipramine (Norpramin)—work on pain from damage to a nerve root caused by disk herniation, surgical trauma, tumors, and pain from spinal cord injury.

Tricyclics are easy to take. Once the proper dosage is found, it does not change over time and one pill once or, with desipramine, twice a day is enough. They can be easily combined with other pain-relieving medication as needed.

Side Effects. Best of all, many people can tolerate at least one of the tricyclics well. They vary in side effects. Elavil is the most sedating and the most likely to cause other side effects, such as dry mouth, urinary retention in men with enlarged prostates, worsening of ocular pressure in glaucoma, heart rhythm problems, a fall in blood pressure when rising from a lying or seated position, occasional sexual dysfunction in men, and, rarely, menstrual irregularities and the production of breast milk. All members of this class can cause weight gain. The more sedating Elavil may be useful in reducing agitation anxiety and may also promote nighttime sleep, not a bad thing for patients with severe pain.

Norpramin has the fewest side effects. It may be more likely to cause insomnia, undisturbing but vivid dreams, and a degree of agitation. I prefer Pamelor to Norpramin for most patients and rarely use Elavil because of the significant sedation and other side effects it has.

Pamelor, which is as effective as Elavil in relieving pain from nerve damage, also promotes sleep in most patients, without morning grogginess—Elavil's side effects—or daytime agitation. Yet, out of tradition more than anything else, most physicians will prescribe Elavil for nerve-related pain instead of the other drugs in this class. If you are offered a prescription for Elavil for nerve-related pain, ask for the same dose of Pamelor.

Selective Serotonin Reuptake Inhibitors

A group of antidepressants called selective serotonin reuptake inhibitors (SSRI), such as Prozac, Paxil, Effexor, Zoloft, and Wellbutrin, is used for all sorts of things: depression, shyness, panic attacks. They appear to be less effective than tricyclic antidepressants in treating pain, but they have fewer major side effects than the older tricyclics. They may cause such problems as weight gain, minor sleep disturbance, and the inability to attain orgasm or ejaculate.

The catch here is that not all antidepressants have good pain-relieving qualities. However, relieving depression and anxiety, both symptoms that commonly accompany chronic pain, also helps to relieve physical pain. If these drugs help depression as well as or better than a tricyclic or are better tolerated, they should by all means be used, possibly in combination with low doses of a tricyclic. By lessening the depression from chronic pain, you may feel better. We need more research to come up with drugs that are effective and well tolerated in treating pain and depression simultaneously.

OTHER NONNARCOTIC DRUGS

Anticonvulsants or antiseizure drugs are used to treat the same sort of pain from nerve damage as the tricyclics. The nervous system is electrical. In a simplified form, neuropathic pain is like a seizure in some nerves—from a short circuit or sparking in "wires" of the nervous system. A seizure is an explosion of electrical activity in overactive brain cells. Pain from a damaged nerve root, spinal cord, or the brain involves inappropriate or overactive firing of nerve cells. Anticonvulsants reduce this abnormal firing.

Phenytoin (Dilantin), carbamazepine (Tegretol), gabapentin (Neurontin), topiramate (Topomax), lamotrigine (Lamictal), and valproic acid (Depakote) are six popular antiseizure medications that treat the pain from irritable or damaged nerves. However, not everyone, especially not the elderly, can tolerate dosages high enough to relieve pain from nervous system damage.

Antiarrhythmics or sodium channel blockers were developed to control abnormal rhythms of the heart. Like the nervous system, the heart is electrical, so these blockers—they include mexiletine (Mexitil) and tocainamide (Tonocard)—can stop the abnormal and painful firing of damaged nerves that control the transmission of pain impulses. These drugs are not without potential cardiac side effects, and they can damage the liver. However, they can usually be used effectively and safely in very low doses, alone or in combination with other pain medication, in the treatment of chronic pain from damaged nerves.

Tramadol (Ultram) is a fairly new painkiller with two separate mechanisms of action. It binds to the same sites on nerves to which the narcotics adhere. It also, like the tricyclic antidepressants, manipulates norepinephrine and serotonin. In spite of its dual action, it is only about as powerful as codeine, which is used for mild-to-moderate pain, such as that seen after some dental procedures. The concept behind this drug—working on more than one pain-controlling system at the same time—is intriguing and may be exploited to better advantage with other drugs in the future.

Ultram is not a narcotic, but because it binds to narcotic receptors on nerve cells in the cord and brain, it acts like one. Theoretically, it may cause addiction in anyone who is predisposed to it. In practice, Ultram addiction is exceedingly rare. Like narcotics, it may cause sleepiness, nausea, and constipation.

MYTHS AND TRUTHS ABOUT USING NARCOTICS FOR BACK PAIN

In 2003, Rush Limbaugh, the conservative radio personality, admitted that he was addicted to his painkillers. He used the narcotic Oxycontin as one of his drugs of abuse. Limbaugh has very real back pain problems. Apparently, he has had spinal surgery and had been seriously overweight. Why and how he became addicted to the drugs is anybody's guess, but he was apparently taking thirty to forty pills a day, which he bought on the black market. I do not know the specifics of his pain predicament nor how and why he became addicted to narcotics. However, with the media attention the drug has received, the fallout from his addiction is considerable.

Oxycontin is a powerful, long-acting, timed-release narcotic that provides pain relief for eight to twelve hours, compared with four hours for a short-acting drug like Percocet. Percocet contains oxycodone, the same narcotic as Oxycontin, combined with acetaminophen (Tylenol), and is used for moderate to severe cancer pain and other types of pain.

Oxycontin was and probably still is being used purely to get high, often with lethal consequences. Users do not take the pill in the manner for which it was intended, giving them a smooth release of the narcotic over a twelve-hour period.

Instead, they crush it and snort it, put it under their tongues, and shoot it up. This intentional bastardization of the pill allows the entire dose of the drug to be released at once. The means by which these addicts deliver it to themselves also permits rapid uptake of the drug into the bloodstream and brain within minutes. According to addicts, this results in a feeling of tremendous power. (In all too many unfortunate cases, it is followed by sleepiness, depressed breathing, and death. This has led various states to begin litigation against the manufacturer.)

Pharmacies carrying the drug have been robbed at gunpoint. A very small group of physicians issued prescriptions of this drug to make money as a drug-issuing mill— to less than credible patients. Since this negative publicity, many physicians, already afraid of creating narcotic addicts, have become even more reluctant to write narcotic prescriptions.

My office administrator, upon hearing about the Limbaugh scandal, insisted that I switch any patient in my practice on Oxycontin to a substitute drug, purely for political reasons. "You don't want to be associated with that mess," she admonished. Of course I didn't do anything of the sort, but her position vividly demonstrates the effect of this Oxycontin debacle even on those sympathetic to the legitimate use of narcotics.

As a physician I must educate the public, my patients, staff, and colleagues about the realities of Oxycontin and other narcotic use and potential abuse and disabuse them of irrational concepts. Does banning such a drug serve the vast majority of patients in chronic moderate-to-severe pain who are not addicts, never become addicts, and require narcotics to have a decent quality of life?

Using Narcotics for Pain Does Not Make You an Addict

People in pain can be treated effectively with narcotics without becoming drug addicts. As head of the Pain Clinic at the Veterans Administration hospital in Manhattan, I met a great patient, Bill Trent, who was able to pull himself out of the quicksand of disability. In a Gulf War battle Bill's spine was injured. A broken vertebra in his lower spine had partially crushed a nerve root in his lower back, numbing and weakening part of his leg and sending excruciating pain down to his left foot. Before I saw him, Bill had had a bone fragment surgically removed from his spine. It was a small fragment, but it was in a bad place. Bill's spine did not become unstable, but he was in chronic pain with short episodes of exacerbation that occurred several times a day. After listening to his history and examining him, I worked out some strategies with Bill to get rid of his pain.

We worked with a host of drugs in various combinations for a few months with good but incomplete benefits. Bill wanted more pain control, but he wanted, if possible, to take less medication.

Using the results from a few diagnostic blocks, we surmised that the tip of his spinal cord or the root near its entry into the cord had been damaged by bone fragments. It was probable that the pain had become "programmed" into his spinal cord and even his brain as a consequence of this type of injury. Abnormal circuits had grown in his cord, perpetuating pain even though there was no external painful sensation causing it. All the blocks in the world would not solve his problem.

Finally, we refined Bill's analgesic regimen until we found one, based on both short- and long-acting morphine, that worked for him. Because Bill is young, he had minimal side effects and they were easy to manage, so it was not difficult to find the correct dosage. However, three years after he came to me, his pain had increased because his body had gotten used to the dosage. I increased it slightly with excellent effect. It didn't even cross my mind that he was acting like an addict, and he certainly wasn't. He is realistic and knows he will have some pain and disability all his life. That nerve root—or spinal cord—will never stop sending sparks to the brain.

He also knows that, for all this problems, he is lucky that it did not affect his bowel, bladder, or sexual function and that he has a supportive wife. Best of all, he has character and will. Knowing that his days of driving a truck were over, Bill went to school to become, of all things, a physical therapist. He has become an extraordinary one and a role model to his patients.

Fear of addiction should not prevent you from seeking pain relief. In a survey published in 1999 that was conducted for the American Academy of Pain Medicine and the American Pain Society, 49 percent of those who had taken narcotic pain relievers said they were concerned about addiction. Yet the data clearly shows that the vast majority of patients with pain do *not* become addicted to narcotics they take.

With appropriate choice of drugs, safeguards, and monitoring of patients, narcotics can be safely and effectively prescribed for moderate-to-severe chronic pain, even in settings where there is an already high population of addicts and alcoholics. I can attest to this from my knowledge of the academic literature and my experience as head of the Pain Clinic at the Manhattan Veterans Administration hospital.

Doctors measure pain as they do other vital signs, such as blood pressure, pulse, and temperature. When pain is treated, it must be monitored, just like following a fever in treating an infection. Doctors who prescribe pain medications without monitoring their patients not only enable inappropriate use of narcotics but are also not likely to maximize the treatment of their patients' pain.

DRUG TOLERANCE, DEPENDENCE, AND ADDICTION

Remember that first cigarette behind the garage? Boy, did it make you green. Your body wasn't used to it. If you were foolish enough to keep smoking, you got used to the effect of nicotine: tolerant of it. You wouldn't turn green and would want to smoke more cigarettes, even feel terrible if you couldn't get any. You had become dependent on nicotine. Worse yet, you craved cigarettes, purely because you liked to smoke or the way smoking made you feel. That is a form of addiction. It is psychological more than physical.

Tolerance means that the body adapts to a narcotic so that it may have both less therapeutic value and fewer side effects. Fortunately, tolerance to the side effects of opiates develops quickly, but tolerance to the pain-relieving effects of these drugs develops slowly, for unclear reasons. Most chronic pain, once controlled, may be treated with a stable dose with little need for more drugs. In practical terms, someone in chronic pain may take the equivalent of four to six Percocets daily for years with good results and few side effects. They get used to the side effects of the drug. A person not used to that amount of narcotic would become sleepy and act as if overdosed. A few people do become tolerant to the pain-relieving properties of a narcotic. If this happens, raising the dosage or changing to another narcotic that interacts differently with the specialized (narcotic sensitive) pain-controlling nerve cells in the brain and spinal cord may help control the pain. This strategy may outwit the mechanism of tolerance. If these therapeutic maneuvers either do not work, or are not tolerated by the patient because of excessive narcotic side effects, intraspinal delivery of narcotic is another option.

Dependence is your body's adaptation to the continued or repeated presence of a drug, such as a narcotic. In the absence of the drug for a period, your body goes into withdrawal. Have you ever seen people in the office who decided to go off caffeine for a while? Why, they can become bears— jittery, headachy; you've seen them. If coffee drinkers go without their drug, they will have withdrawal symptoms, just like the withdrawal symptoms from other substances, including narcotics.

Dependence and tolerance are normal physiological adaptations to the regular exposure of the central nervous system—and the body—to a chemical. If Bill the truck driver were to stop taking his narcotics, he would go into withdrawal. But he never uses narcotics to get high. He uses them for pain.

Addiction is using a drug for psychological purposes: to get high. Addicts are truly different from nonaddicts. For example, it has been shown that there is at least a partial genetic predisposition toward addiction for both drug use and alcohol, illustrating the possibility of addicts' biological uniqueness. Addiction to and abuse of prescribed narcotics occurs in about the same percentage of people as become alcoholics or engage in other substance abuse. Addicts report euphoria from narcotic use; most nonaddicts report either no change in their psychological state or a mildly disagreeable feeling. Drugs to an addict are an end unto themselves.

HOW TO USE NARCOTICS EFFECTIVELY

The amount of narcotic given (dose) and method of giving it (delivery) depend on many things, including the severity and nature of the pain and the pain-relieving and side effects of the drug. The beneficial effect of a narcotic depends on its potency, how much gets to the pain-modulating nerve cells of the spinal cord, which keep pain impulses from causing you to feel or react to pain. Obviously, the duration of the pain-relieving action is important, too. Its side effects depend in part on how much drug arrives in the brain (sedation) and bowel (constipation) as well as individual tolerance for a narcotic.

Strength and Delivery Method

For any given drug, the more severe the pain, the more is required to treat it. The strengths and pain-relieving potencies of narcotics vary greatly. Doctors prescribing these drugs take cognizance of these differences when choosing doses or switching from one narcotic to another. Just as scotch is stronger than sherry, oxycodone, the narcotic in Percocet, is twice as strong as morphine. So twice as much morphine as Percocet is needed for the same effect.

Drug delivery deals with the mechanism controlling two things: the amount of narcotic that gets to the pain-controlling nerve cells and how fast it gets there. When you swallow a pill, it takes about forty-five minutes to be absorbed and digested. Some of the narcotic in the pill is destroyed by the digestive process before it reaches the brain and spinal cord, so less is available to diminish pain. This delivery method also causes constipation because of the effect of the local effect of the narcotic on the gastrointestinal system.

One of the advantages of the Duragesic skin patch is that the narcotic, fentanyl, is delivered through the skin into the fat under the skin and eventually into the tiny blood vessels in that fat. From there it goes directly to the central nervous system, bypassing the digestive system. The patch allows more narcotic to be delivered to the spinal cord, so you get pain relief with less constipation. Administration of narcotics by a skin patch into the fat under the skin, subcutaneously, intravenously, or intraspinally delivers relatively more narcotic into the cord with less constipation. Unlike pills, these methods all bypass the digestive system.

Intravenous delivery gets the narcotic to the spinal cord faster than a pill or a patch. It is more efficient than patches but also more invasive. When needed, it's worth it.

Intraspinal injection of morphine allows still less narcotic to be given with fewer side effects than any of the above means. More invasive, it is required to adequately control some acute and chronic pain with acceptable side effects. Intraspinal injection of a given dose of narcotic may give ten to a hundred times more pain relief than the same dose intravenously. The variability in effect from an intraspinal dose depends on whether the narcotic is delivered into the epidural space or spinal fluid (intrathecally). However, with any form of intraspinal delivery, the drug is delivered close to its site of action: the spinal cord nerve cells in which narcotics modulate or inhibit pain transmission from body to brain. Less of the drug is delivered to the brain and bowels, so side effects are less severe.

In hospitalized patients, epidural infusions of pain medication, usually combined with a PCA pump, may be briefly used to control acute postoperative pain. In patients with chronic pain, intraspinal analgesia is provided with a refillable pump, buried under the skin from which a plastic tube carries the medication from the pump to the spinal fluid in the upper lumbar region.

Whether the pain is acute or chronic, the rate of pain relief required to treat it is important in choosing a means of delivery. For chronic pain or mild-to-moderate acute pain, pills or patches make sense. The right dose and schedule for using the pills can be determined over a few days. Once the correct dose and method for taking them is determined, you can take them for long periods with good results. *Severe* acute pain must be addressed more quickly, within minutes.

Scheduling Narcotic Medications

The duration of pain relief provided by a particular drug must relate to the problem being treated. Severe chronic back pain requires around-the-clock narcotic coverage with longer-acting drugs, possibly supplemented with short-acting drugs. Some preparations last from three to four hours (morphine), eight to twelve hours (MS Contin, Oxycontin, Kadian), or twenty-four hours (Avinza, Kadian). Fentanyl skin patches (Duragesic) last three days in most people, but in some only two to two and a half days.

Awareness of the duration of a drug's action leads to good pain control with few side effects. In younger people, Kadian may have to be given every twelve hours. Giving it once a day may not control pain. In older people, once-a-day may work; Kadian twice a day may make them sleepy.

Side Effects

Use of narcotics may cause many side effects: nausea, vomiting, constipation, sleepiness, sweating, mild mental clouding, loss of appetite, loss of libido, to name a few. With long-term treatment, most people become tolerant of most narcotic side effects within a week or two, except constipation, which usually has to be treated over a long term.

Combining Different Types of Drugs

In many difficult-to-control pain states, drugs can be used in combination. You may need a long-acting narcotic and a short-acting one plus another drug to work more specifically on pain from damaged nerves and one or several drugs to control the side effects of the narcotics (most commonly constipation).

To treat a chronically painful back, a narcotic can be combined with NSAIDs or acetaminophen (Tylenol) to achieve better pain relief with less narcotic and fewer narcotic side effects. Narcotics and NSAIDs act on different pain-relieving mechanisms. As it turns out, adding an NSAID to a narcotic has a synergistic effect, which is more than an additive effect. In other words, synergy might be two plus two equals six; an additive effect is two plus two equals four.

Prozac and similar antidepressants can accelerate the metabolism or breakdown of narcotics. Patients using these may require larger or more frequent doses of narcotics, not because they are depressed drug addicts but because the narcotics don't last as long.

Why the Effects Vary

We all experience pain and react differently to the effects and side effects of narcotics. Those of us who experience more pain or require more narcotics aren't necessarily either wimps or addicts. Some people break down narcotics faster than others. Ten percent of the population derives no significant pain relief from codeine because of their body's inability to process the drug usefully. In terms of side effects, some patients will tolerate one narcotic poorly and another without a problem.

The most common form of intolerance to a narcotic is severe nausea. Sometimes there is vomiting also. These are not manifestations of a drug allergy; they just mean that you don't tolerate that narcotic. Intolerance to morphine, for example, doesn't mean you are intolerant of such sister drugs as oxycodone or other classes of narcotics.

I was asked to evaluate an elderly women who was in terrible pain from osteoporotic fractures of her spine and ribs. She had been on corticosteroids for years because of a rheumatological disease and had severe osteoporosis. She was in so much pain in my office that she couldn't sit or lie down, in spite of her oral narcotics: Percocet and Oxycontin. I immediately sent her to the hospital and started her on an intravenous morphine infusion. (There is no intravenous form of oxycodone, the narcotic in the tablets she was taking.) In spite of drugs to suppress nausea, the morphine made her retch so badly that she broke more ribs. So I switched her to an infusion of another narcotic—Dilaudid—and it worked like a charm. The next day when I saw her, she asked me why I was keeping her in the hospital now that her pain was gone!

This story illustrates why I am in favor of more, not fewer, narcotics, on the market. They all may be effective, but some patients who need them cannot tolerate most of them. Getting around their side effects and maximizing pain control is helped by a wider, not a narrower, spectrum of narcotics from which to choose. Those antiaddiction zealots who want Oxycontin taken off the market and to slow the introduction of new narcotics should realize the disservice these policies have on the millions of legitimate chronic pain patients who require narcotics to live a decent life.

Timing the Doses

Timing medicine correctly is as important as finding the correct one. If you know a pill takes forty-five minutes to work, don't wait until your back hurts to take it. Anticipate what you are going to do and take it before you take a walk, play with the kids, or go shopping so that the medicine will have taken effect when the pain starts. This will also keep your dosage down. If a medication works for four hours, watch the clock. Be aware that after three and a half hours, you should take it again. Otherwise, you are going to have pain in the middle of your Christmas shopping spree and will squirm until the pill takes effect. I urge my patients to avoid the seesaw of taking medicine and having it wear off. Most narcotics with which you are familiar (codeine, Vicodin, Percocet, and morphine) last only four hours, not six, as they are usually prescribed.

Relief of chronic back pain can take time, and it requires communication, trust, and patience between doctor and patient. For example, of the drugs I have mentioned, it may take two months to arrive at the proper dosage of Neurontin: if the dose is raised too quickly, severe sleepiness may occur. Anticonvulsants like Dilantin and Tegretol can take at least two weeks to adjust. Tricyclics like Pamelor or Elavil may also take a week or two. That is a fairly short period but not to a person who is suffering through side effects and waiting for pain relief.

BALANCING RELIEF AND SIDE EFFECTS

In evaluating what kinds of side effects are acceptable, you have to weigh what is wrong with you, what medications and procedures can help you, and what the chances are that your condition will improve on its own or is instead chronic.

Severe nausea and vomiting are not acceptable side effects when beginning narcotics, but a few days of queasiness is. Most patients get used to the majority of narcotic side effects in a week, except for constipation, which will not go away but can be treated with a high-fiber diet, lots of fluids, stool softener, and possibly a laxative. It is not acceptable to be drowsy or so sedated that you walk like a drunk. If as a result of a new drug regimen you are sleepy for a few hours of the day and also have a 75 percent reduction of chronic severe otherwise intractable back pain that you had for years, the benefits of pain relief surely outweigh the side effects. That's how doctors weigh side effects. It's common sense.

The most serious side effect of narcotics—the slowing of respiration and buildup of deadly carbon dioxide from inadequate breathing—is rare if they are used as prescribed. Obviously, if someone wants to commit suicide by taking all his Percocet at once, he could succeed—or end up with brain damage from severe narcotic-induced depression of respiratory function.

The trick is to find the least invasive way of getting the best pain relief with the fewest, least severe side effects. Careful trial and error with several different drugs can very often achieve excellent pain control with few and minor side effects without having to resort to invasive methods. Indeed, the vast majority of patients can be treated with pills or, possibly, a patch.

Practical Issues

The initial choice of prescribing one narcotic over another is often based on a physician's experience. If he or she is more used to prescribing morphine than oxycodone, that is what will be used first if all other things are equal, such as the patient's previous response to the drug or its cost.

Key Points about Medication for Pain
- Pain can be minimized even if its underlying cause cannot be cured.
- Taking narcotics to control pain does not in most cases lead to addiction.
- Taking pain medication does not mean you are a weakling.

- Controlling your pain quickly and efficiently preserves your sense of well-being, your lifestyle, and your livelihood.
- Most doctors do not prescribe adequate pain medication, so patients suffer unnecessarily.
- You may need to try a variety of narcotic drugs to find one that works for you.

Chapter 18

Radiofrequency Lesioning and Other Interventional Treatment for Back Pain

It is always wise to begin any treatment conservatively then if necessary work up the ladder of invasiveness. If rest, hot compresses, medications, and physical therapy isn't working or is inappropriate, there are a variety of techniques to relieve back pain, some using drugs, that may be appropriate. These include epidural injections, nerve and facet blocks, radiofrequency lesioning, IDET, laser therapy, vertebroplasty, and implanted devices.

EPIDURAL STEROID INJECTIONS

Epidural injections can relieve the pain from a new disk herniation, a tear in the disk cover, mild-to-moderate stenosis, or, after surgery, pain from an inflamed, swollen nerve root. They may help while the disk or root is given time to heal on its own. The steroid is injected into the fatty space within the spinal canal to bathe the nerve roots with medication. One of the reasons we have pain when nerve roots are pressed by a disk herniation is that nerves under pressure become swollen. They expand against whatever is already pressing on them, such as a piece of disk, making the pressure worse and increasing the pain. Some remain swollen and cause pain for a while even after the pressure is removed. This explains some bouts of postoperative pain, even with a good surgical decompression (removal of pressure on the roots).

Theoretically, steroids reduce swelling within the root, causing it to shrink. This reduces the pressure on it and thus reduces the pain impulses that are generated. Besides acting on the swollen nerves, the liquid in the epidural also flushes away the body's chemicals produced by disk herniations or annular tears that cause root inflammation and more nerve root pain.

Most physicians combine the steroid injection with local anesthetic, and a few even use a bit of narcotic to give you immediate relief. In people with tight spinal canals from congenital or acquired stenosis, the amount of liquid injected with the epidural may increase the pressure on the roots, causing more pain for a few hours. The beneficial steroid effect doesn't begin for a day or so.

Epidurals are purely therapeutic, unlike diagnostic blocks, and epidural local anesthetic is not without some risk (see below). Therefore, I do not use local anesthetic in epidurals on elderly patients with acquired stenosis. I do not use local anesthetic in epidurals on elderly patients with acquired stenosis. However, I select patients so they do quite well, experiencing little pain with my technique. Also, the vast majority of stenosis patients I treat with epidurals (frequently combined with root blocks) usually have complicated spines, with multiple areas of stenosis pressing on nerve roots and causing symptoms (see Chapter 12). These patients are given epidurals not in the office but in an outpatient or hospital radiological facility. They get a mild intravenous anesthesia, and the procedure is accurately performed using a CT scanner or fluoroscopy.

Should You Have an Epidural?

Epidurals are both used and abused in the management of chronic pain, so it's a good idea to understand in whom they are effective. Remember, the injection is meant to make you feel better, not for just a few days but for the long term.

Epidurals work best for a very small specific group of people, such as those under forty with pain from disk herniation and tears in the disk cover who have not previously had surgery or those with pain lasting less than three months. For the long term, they do not relieve the radicular leg pain due to nerve root irritation from a herniated disk or reduce the need for eventual surgery. The same presumably applies to cervical-disk herniations.

Epidurals can be useful in treating postoperative nerve-root-related pain but only if there is no residual pressure on the painful root, that is, if the surgeon has fully decompressed the painful root. They can be useful for short-term pain relief from mild-to-moderate stenosis, but they don't give significant long-term relief.

Epidurals are not helpful for localized neck or back pain from painful facets, even though they are often misused for this symptom.

In the long run, epidurals do not work well as substitutes for adequate surgery to decompress nerve roots.

There are no good scientific studies demonstrating the superiority of oral to epidural steroids for disk herniations, annulus tears, nerve-root pain after surgery, or stenosis. However, I tend to use short courses of oral steroids where possible, because they are often effective and are less risky than the more invasive epidural injections. When patients have had unsuccessful epidurals performed without radiological guidance, I may suggest a radiologically guided injection to insure good coverage of all areas of nerve-root compression by the steroid solution. If the guided injections don't work, despite good coverage of the roots with steroids, you know that further injections are useless.

I may use epidurals instead of oral steroids in patients who for medical reasons should not use oral steroids. Those who have already had one or two courses of oral steroids with good results and are getting better but still need some steroids to help them through their recovery may be good candidates for epidurals. I rarely use them for patients who were not helped by oral steroids. If oral steroids don't work, epidurals usually won't work either.

Risks

If you are taking a blood thinner like Coumadin, you should not have an epidural because it may result in massive bleeding or permanent nerve damage.

Accidental puncture of the dura and arachnoid covering the spinal cord and nerve roots may result in giving the injection into the spinal fluid. This can be life-threatening if not managed properly. Steroids injected into the spinal fluid—even without local anesthetic—have produced a progressive scarring of the arachnoid in a small number of people (see Chapter 1). This scar may squeeze the nerves and spinal cord covered by the arachnoid, resulting in progressive numbness, weakness, and pain. Rarely, bowel and bladder dysfunction may occur.

Puncturing the dura and arachnoid may also cause chronic leakage of spinal fluid into the epidural space through the hole produced by the needle. Normally, the hole closes up; when it doesn't, it can leak whenever you sit or stand. This may cause a spinal headache, which usually diminishes with bedrest, painkillers, and taking in lots of fluids. If conservative therapy doesn't help in a few days, a small amount of your blood can be injected into the epidural space to form a clot and patch the hole.

The risk of puncturing the dura and arachnoid is greater if you have stenosis, large disk herniation, stenosis, or have had surgery at the site of the epidural. Epidurals given in previously operated-on locations should be performed with radiological guidance.

Local anesthetic placed properly into the epidural space blocks the sympathetic nerves that control blood pressure. The body usually responds quickly to this block to minimize a possible drop in blood pressure. In some situations, however, blood pressure can drop precipitously, requiring IV fluids and medication. This is more likely to occur in the elderly, people with high blood pressure, those on some heart medications, diabetics, and patients with moderate-to-severe stenosis.

Rarely injections in the epidural space can occur following an epidural. An abscess in the space may form and require surgical drainage of the area quickly to prevent damage to the cord or roots compressed by the abscess. Rarely a cervical or thoracic epidural needle will not only pierce the dura and arachnoid, but also the spinal cord. I have seen two patients with this problem despite fluoroscopy-guided epidurals. One recovered fully and the other was left with a mild permanent weakness and numbness of the arm.

The benefit of epidurals and other procedures I've talked about are real. So are the risk and costs. Make sure the benefits are worth it to you, and the physician performing them is highly experienced.

FACET AND NERVE-ROOT BLOCKS

Local anesthetics alone or mixed with corticosteroids can also be injected into the spinal facets or over the nerves carrying pain impulses from them. These nerves are branches of larger ones that control the muscles and skin of the neck and back. Other targets for these injections are the nerve roots exiting the spine. Beyond the purview of this book, they can be injected outside the spine over peripheral nerves. These injections are called facet, branch, root, or nerve blocks, respectively.

Unlike epidurals, most of these blocks should be used primarily as diagnostic tools (see Chapter 3) with possible therapeutic effects. (For some disk herniations off to one side of the spine, a block through the foramen under radiological guidance—which is how a root block is performed—may be the best way to deposit steroids for therapeutic purposes into the epidural space on a compressed root.) Whatever therapeutic effect such injections may have usually diminishes with time. Just like the injections from your rheumatologist or orthopedist, they wear off in a few months or less. Your pain usually returns once their effects have waned.

The important question about blocks is what to do if they work then wear off or if they don't work at all. What is Plan B? More blocks? For how long and to what end? Ending up married to a "block doc" who, over the long term, simply repeats blocks that last only a few weeks or a few months makes little sense from your point of view. You need to find a treatment that effectively ends your pain.

Blocks paid for by low-paying insurers are often performed quickly and inaccurately, with incomplete coverage of the pain generators. It is simply not cost effective for physicians in some plans to take the time to perform these blocks perfectly. Many if not most insurance companies impose limits on the number of blocks you can have in one year, often three at the most. If you need six, you'll have to live on medication with lifestyle reduction and some degree of chronic pain. Or you'll have to pay for a big part of your treatment out of pocket.

Clearly the diagnostic accuracy of these injections is important. Facet pain usually comes from several facets: often four to six. For the blocks to relieve pain temporarily, all of the painful facets must be identified, from clinical history and findings. If painful facets are not accurately injected, the pain emanating from them will not be relieved. You and the physician may then conclude that the facets are not the principal source of pain. Moreover, if the blocks are not accurate, the local anesthetic destined for the facet or its nerves may spill onto nearby structures, such as the spinal root in the foramen, and an inadvertent root block will thereby be performed. This may give misleading diagnostic data. The physician may think the facet is the pain-generator when in fact the root or disk covering may be. Performing a radiofrequency lesion of the nerves to the facets based on incorrect data will waste the patient's time and money and not relieve his or her pain.

Doctors Who Perform Nerve and Facet Blocks

Nerve and facet blocks should be performed by a skilled physician who has significant experience in this area. Weekend courses are given to physicians to get them acquainted with various procedures, such as diagnostic blocks, radiofrequency lesions, and IDET. You do not want to be the Monday-morning patient of a doctor who just returned from one of these courses. Blocks in spinal structures should be done with high-quality X-ray guidance to safely and accurately place the needle correctly and verify the placement of the injected liquids.

Unfortunately, these blocks are just as overused by pain-management specialists as fusions are overused by spine surgeons, EMGs by neurologists, and physical therapy by physiatrists.

Be sure that you have a nerve block done by an experienced physician who is diagnostically and technically skilled and still has a traditional style of practice, one in which he or she can provide a complete diagnostic evaluation. Blocks may help confirm a diagnosis that was based on a thorough evaluation, including your history, physical exam, and radiological and other tests. Diagnostic blocks should not be used to make a diagnosis. Normally, you should not have repeated therapeutic blocks instead of medication, more definitive pain-relieving procedures, or surgery. Remember the Plan B issue.

CUTTING OFF THE PAIN IMPULSE: RADIOFREQUENCY LESIONING

Radiofrequency energy can be used to achieve highly selective complete or partial destruction of the nerves that carry pain impulses. These nerves may be carrying pain from facets, disks, nerve roots themselves, or areas of the body sending impulses up the peripheral nerves to specific nerve roots and eventually to the cord and brain. The energy is delivered through a thin electrode placed in the body over a specific nerve or nerves. Such a destruction of nerves is called a lesion, meaning wound or injury. The extent of intentional nerve damage depends on the nerve that is being lesioned. Some nerves can tolerate more of a lesion than others without incurring side effects. The trick is to know which nerves to damage for a given pain problem.

Long-Term Pain Relief

Radiofrequency lesioning is a highly effective, safe, proven treatment for chronic pain, one that provides years of relief. If you have not benefited from standard conservative therapy for spinal pain, some radiofrequency procedures provide at least eighteen months of significant—at least a 50 percent reduction—relief of pain without using more pain medication than was used before the lesioning or forcing changes in lifestyle. The amount of pain medication is usually reduced and activity level increased, and the patient experiences significant pain reduction after successful treatment with this technique. The goal of pain therapy is to restore function and reduce the need for medication.

Studies have shown that neck and head pain coming from cervical spinal structures may be significantly reduced in more than 80 percent of patients. Similarly, pain in the lower shoulders, between the shoulder blades, and in the spine behind the ribs may be significantly reduced in 90 percent of patients. Finally, low-back and related buttock, hip, groin, thigh, and upper leg pain may be significantly reduced in at least 45 percent of patients (in my experience, it is closer to 65 percent). These techniques—usually in the form of ganglion lesions—have been applied to patients with spine-related pain from cancer with good, lasting results. The ganglion is the sensory computer, or relay station, of a nerve root that sends pain impulses from a peripheral nerve to the spinal cord and on to the brain. These lesions cut down the number of pain signals traveling along the nerve to the spinal cord and eventually the brain. I have used ganglion lesions in the treatment of such diverse problems as headaches, painful groins from hernia operations, and spinal pain in some cancer patients with lasting results. I have also used radiofrequency lesions of the disks to treat painful disks, with 70 percent of patients reporting greater than 75 percent relief of pain within a week and lasting well over two years. Finally, benign painful bone tumors can be eradicated with radiofrequency lesions with the same success rate as open surgery. This technique is increasingly used in some large hospitals to treat these tumors.

Radiofrequency lesions at the appropriate sites in and around the spine, performed accurately by an experienced physician, are safe and effective and should have no permanent side effects. If they are successful but the benefit wears off over several years because the nerves grew back, they can be repeated with good results. If they don't work, go on to other therapy.

How It Works

Local anesthesia is applied to the skin and muscles. In my practice, an anesthesiologist administers intravenous sedating medication and, at the moment of lesioning, intravenous pain medication. One of a series of lesions is made in one procedure, which in my practice takes forty-five to ninety minutes. Heat emanates from an ultrathin electrode that is connected to a specialized radiofrequency generator. The electrode, insulated except at the tip, is accurately placed with fluoroscopic or CT guidance through the skin and muscles, terminating over the nerves to a particular facet, in a painful disk, or over the ganglion.

Inaccuracy of even a few millimeters in electrode placement is enough for the target nerve to escape adequate lesioning or for nearby structures to be damaged. Inaccuracy can damage a root, the spinal cord, or an artery to the cord or brain, and structures around the spine with possibly temporary or permanent consequences.

Once the positioning is verified, depending on the particular nerve, it is heated for 90 to 120 seconds to around 160 to 175 degrees Fahrenheit. Multiple lesions in painful disks are made at 175 degrees for several minutes. Lesions are made at different locations within the disk. For the ganglia or nerves supplying the facets, local anesthetic is placed through the electrode to anesthetize the nerve and surrounding area before making the lesion. This is not necessary for lesions within the disk, which are well tolerated with the help of a little intravenous pain medication.

This technique can safely, selectively, and effectively lesion the ganglion without damaging the root or nearby structures. Radiolesioning can provide good sustained pain relief in well-chosen patients. When performed properly, the treatment does not seriously damage any nerves other than those lesioned.

You can go home thirty to sixty minutes after the procedure. (You can't drive until the intravenous medication wears off.)

The nerves that supply the facet joint can be destroyed this way. However, the treatment cannot erase the cause of the pain: facet-joint degeneration. Nor does it do anything to halt disk degeneration.

After the Procedure

Correctly performed procedures using the above techniques may cause increased pain around the lesioned area for several weeks, but I have never met a patient who could not go to work the day after the lesions (possibly with the help of pain relievers).

In some patients, lesions may result, for fewer than three months, in patchy numbness or mild supersensitivity of the skin of the back controlled by the lesioned nerves. This is especially true when lesioning facets in the uppermost neck or a ganglion. Even when the procedure is done properly, not all the sources of pain may be reached: facets may not be the whole story. Fifty percent reduction of pain in the long term is considered a good outcome. Patients often ask me if they can hurt themselves by overdoing it after a successful radiofrequency treatment. No. If they overdo it and herniate a disk or fall and break a facet, they will of course experience severe pain, but in practical terms, they cannot hurt their arthritic facet joints merely by having a more active physical existence, either.

The lesioned nerves may eventually grow back and pain may recur. Fortunately, for most people, pain does not recur in the lesioned area. If necessary, you can be re-treated with radiofrequency lesioning with excellent long-term results.

Doctors Who Perform Radiofrequency Lesioning: What They Do and Don't Do

Radiofrequency lesioning technique, as applied to the nervous system, dates back to the 1950s, when it was developed by neurosurgeons for lesioning the brain and cord; by the 1970s, it was being utilized in the treatment of lumbar spine pain. In the late 1980s and 1990s, it was applied with great success to pain conditions in the cervical and thoracic spine. It has repeatedly been shown to be highly effective and safe when performed by skilled physicians, not one who just took a weekend course in the technique. (See Chapter 3 for more information.)

A small but troubling minority of physicians inadvertently damage the wrong nerves or incorrectly lesion the targeted nerves. The net result is no relief and possibly new pain, weakness, or numbness—sometimes permanent—in a leg or arm. Partially in response to this problem, an important supplier of radiofrequency equipment created a generator that permitted low-temperature lesions. These lesions would not cause serious nerve damage but could relieve pain, although not for nearly as long a period as using the heat technique described above. The traditional heat-based method gives by far the longest duration of pain relief.

Most physicians in this country do not feel it is safe to lesion the ganglia, preferring to implant spinal-cord stimulators or implantable intraspinal pumps before they resort to a ganglion lesion—if they consider using it at all. They fear they'll cause more nerve-related pain after lesioning the ganglion, not to mention permanent weakness and numbness. Alternatively, some now do use the low-temperature method described above for ganglion lesions.

My own experience, and that of many European physicians who described their results with ganglion lesions in respected medical journals, demonstrates the success and safety of ganglion lesions in the right situation. Like any kind of procedure, it has to be performed by the right physician on the appropriate patient to have a reasonable expectation of good results. Find a physician who has considerable experience with conventional, high-temperature ganglion lesions with proven good results before allowing this procedure to be performed on you. In the appropriate situation, lesioning a ganglion is preferable to being married to an implantable device.

Many physicians are also reluctant to apply radiofrequency technique to pain problems in the upper neck or even the thoracic spine, because in these locations there is a greater possibility of creating inadvertent damage to the lung, spinal cord, or arteries supplying the brain. Yet they may tell you only that you are not a candidate for radiofrequency lesioning, not that you are not a candidate in their hands.

SIMILAR TECHNIQUES

Techniques similar to radiofrequency lesioning, such as laser therapy, intradiskal radiofrequency, and IDET—intradiskal electrothermal lysis—are also used to treat back pain. There are risks common to all three techniques, although infection or nerve damage occurs in fewer than six disks in a thousand injections. However, I have seen patients whose nerves have been damaged, possibly permanently, through the misplacement of the probe. One of the rare but serious complications of any procedure in which the integrity of the disk is violated by a foreign body is infection.

Laser Therapy for Lumbar Discogenic Pain

Lasers have been used to treat painful disks since the late 1980s. Early studies indicated that 70 percent to 80 percent of patients with lumbar discogenic pain treated by this method had good to excellent improvement. In laser treatment, a small pencil-like object, the laser probe, is inserted into the disk in a way similar to the radiofrequency electrode above except that it is much larger. With some local anesthesia, it is placed under sterile conditions using fluoroscopy, a "live" X-ray that takes continuous images of the physician placing a probe into the body. The nucleus of the disk is then treated with laser energy for a short period, and the probe is removed. Recovery takes a few days.

The proponents of this technique contend that they make a vacuum within the disk so that the nucleus sucks in the disk protrusion, making it less painful. I have never understood how a vacuum can be created in a disk that has a hole in it—an annular tear—from a pencil-sized probe. I feel that the heat from the laser lesions some of the intradiskal nerves, thus reducing the pain. The popularity of this technique waned as IDET became more popular.

Intradiskal Radiofrequency Lesions

In this technique, radiofrequency energy is delivered into the nucleus to treat discogenic pain. The manner in which I use this technique is to insert two or three radiofrequency probes into a disk. The probes are used to make a series of prolonged lesions from the front and center of the disk to the back and sides of it. (Earlier attempts to use a single intradiskal radiofrequency lesion by one probe failed to demonstrate a beneficial effect.) I use CT guidance to carry out this procedure safely and accurately.

Like all procedures that invade the disk, this procedure is performed in a highly sterile manner. Short-acting intravenous and local anesthesia is used to maximize patient comfort.

The procedure takes an hour or two, depending on the location and number of the disk or disks being lesioned. It is performed similarly to other radiofrequency procedures. It may be used for lumbar discogenic pain and is the only technique that can be applied to cervical discogenic pain. The radiofrequency procedure is effective. As mentioned above, 70 percent of patients I have treated with this technique have good to excellent pain relief. You should feel relief quickly and be able to resume your normal lifestyle in a few days. The benefit from the procedure should last over two years. As I describe it, this procedure is not used by other physicians.

Using radiofrequency lesions to treat discogenic pain fell out of favor because previous techniques were ineffective in treating discogenic pain and because IDET (see below) swept the country—prematurely, as you will see. I persisted in using radiofrequency with various modifications and developed the technique outlined above. I have found it very useful. The effect of radiofrequency intradiskal lesions is seen within a day following the procedure and may be applied to disks anywhere in the spine.

The risks of this technique are similar to those for laser treatment of discogenic pain. The small size of the radiofrequency probe makes the risk of disk damage less than with the larger laser or even IDET probes. Unlike radiofrequency, IDET takes several months to work.

In the long run, this radiofrequency technique, like all therapies, needs to be evaluated in a strictly controlled academic study to determine its role in the treatment of discogenic pain.

Dan Ford, thirty-six, is a Wall Street bond trader. He had lumbar disk surgery for the relief of left-leg sciatica with an excellent result until the spontaneous occurrence of excruciating low back pain two weeks before he consulted me. An MRI by his former doctor revealed an annular tear and a significant disk protrusion at the level above the surgical site. Since he didn't require surgery, he was told to stay in bed and take medication. After two weeks he was no better and had not been able to work. His pain disturbed his sleep and plagued him all day long, receding only partially when he was flat on his back.

Dan had three small children to support and, given the nature of his business, was concerned about his income and job future. He was referred to me. I concurred that his pain was probably from the torn annulus, although his MRI suggested that the disk below, which had been operated on, might also be a good candidate for the cause of the pain. There was a suggestion that his spine may also have been unstable at the level of the previous surgery, another cause of pain that could ultimately lead to a reoperation and fusion. X-rays demonstrated that his spine was stable. A discogram revealed that only the disk with the annular tear was the cause of his pain. He was ultimately treated with the radiofrequency disk/annulus heating procedure. In three days he was back to work with no pain. Because of the weakened, protruding disk, Dan had to avoid lifting, bending, and turning of his lower spine to avoid a full disk herniation, which might require further surgery. At work his colleagues commented on how freely he moved, with no facial expression that suggested discomfort. He required no medication and has done well in the two years since the procedure.

IDET

IDET (intradiskal electrothermal lysis) uses conductive heat, like that emitted from a toaster, to treat disk-related pain. Based on small preliminary studies, it was expected that 70 percent of those treated for lumbar discogenic pain would have a good to excellent outcome.

Under sterile conditions, using fluoroscopic guidance and local anesthesia, a wirelike device similar to the heating coil used in a toaster or hair dryer is threaded carefully into the offending disk or disks. The interior of the disk and the part of the annulus facing the spinal canal is heated for about fifteen minutes, after which the wire is removed. It is theorized that this technique lesions the nerves in the overlying annulus and changes the chemical structure of the disk for the better, eventually making it stronger. With this improvement, pain subsides. The IDET procedure may take two to three months of recovery. Indeed, for a while after the procedure, the preexisting pain may temporarily increase.

IDET became popular before it was rigorously evaluated. In one small study in 2000, IDET was evaluated as treatment for discogenic pain. At one year following treatment, 60 percent of those that underwent it had over 50 percent reduction in pain. For various good reasons, data from small studies often indicate superior treatment outcome when compared with large, well-controlled studies.

Well-designed, large studies must be conducted to determine the relative efficacy and limitations of all techniques to control discogenic pain, including fusion, the surgical alternative. The initial enthusiasm for IDET among my colleagues has waned considerably over the last two years. It certainly has not lived up to its early promise. This may be due in part to lack of experience by the physicians who select the patients for the technique and perform it. Like radiofrequency lesions of facets, many weekend courses were given to introduce IDET to pain-management physicians and orthopedic surgeons. This is not to say that IDET or the other treatments don't work or that one is definitely better than the others. The question is in which patients does which therapy work and which physician is able to select them and technically master the treatment technique to be used.

CRYOANALGESIA

For spinal pain, cryoanalgesia is becoming a historical artifact. Cryoanalgesia uses cold instead of heat to create less of a lesion; it results in less nerve destruction than traditional, high-temperature radiofrequency. Like low-temperature radiofrequency, which some physicians employ, cryoanalgesia causes a low-temperature minor reversible lesion. Cryoanalgesia can be used safely to create lesions to control pain transmitted by some peripheral nerves. High-temperature radiofrequency would damage those same nerves, causing more pain, numbness, and sometimes weakness. However, lesions made with this technique last only approximately three months and may need to be repeated.

Aside from the short duration of its effect, the cryoprobe—the device that enters the body to make the lesion—

is about as thick as a pencil, while a radiofrequency probe is thinner than a standard hypodermic needle. Bulky cryoprobes have been used successfully to treat painful lumbar facets but cannot easily be used for lesions in the cervical and thoracic spine, where the anatomical structures are smaller than in the lumbar spine.

Because of the size of the probe and the short-lived effect of cryolesions, this technique can't compete with the utility and effectiveness of the traditional radiofrequency technique for lesioning nerves around the spine. I know of no patients receiving cryolesions for spinal problems anymore, but it is still used for some peripheral nerve pain.

VERTEBROPLASTY

In vertebroplasty, liquefied bone cement is injected through a needle into the collapsed bone. The liquid begins to harden in ten to thirty minutes and stabilizes the bone. This keeps the bone from further collapse and, based on studies, in more than half of cases significantly reduces or gets rid of the pain. The procedure is normally carried out under intravenous anesthesia, using a CT scanner or special X-ray machine called a fluoroscopy unit to guide the doctor in the placement of a needle and the injection of the cement into the weakened bone. There is a 5 percent risk that the cement will leak out of the bone as it is injected, causing potentially serious complications by pressing on the nerves in or around the spine or traveling to blood vessels in the lungs. Most leaks to date have had few serious long-term consequences and required no treatment. Vertebroplasty has been successfully used since 1987, and reports of its benefits and safety in over two hundred patients has been published by various authors in the medical literature.

Vertebroplasty has been used successfully and safely in

the treatment of painful osteoporotic vertebral compression fractures and cancerous tumors that invaded the spine. It has also been vastly overutilized in osteoporotic patients; they would do as well on medication and conservative care. Keep that in mind if it is suggested. Determine through your observations and questions that a less-invasive approach has been tried before considering vertebroplasty. Some 90 percent to 95 percent of patients with osteopororotic vertebral compression fractures do well a few weeks to a few months without vertebroplasty, provided their pain is well controlled with narcotics and other medication. Leave any doctor who offers you vertebroplasty instead of trying hard to treat you with such a medical regimen, even if you have to try several different narcotics until one or (as often happens) a combination is found that you tolerate and works well for you.

Cancer patients may benefit from vertebroplasty as part of a wide-ranging treatment regimen that includes high doses of narcotics and anticancer therapy. It can significantly improve the quality of life of those with metastatic cancer.

IMPLANTABLE DEVICES

Implantable devices, such as spinal cord stimulators and pumps for infusing medication into the spine, have a role in the treatment of severe chronic pain of spinal origin. When used appropriately, they are quite helpful for a small select group of patients who really need them, and for whom nothing else is effective or tolerated. They are never to be used as a substitute for an ongoing noninvasive pain regimen, though they often are. They are also not a substitute for adequate spinal surgery, even though they are, as the case of Myrna illustrates in Chapter 4. Radiofrequency lesions of painful spinal structures should be tried before marrying a patient to a stimulator or pump. These devices implantable under the skin often need adjustment in the physician's office; they periodically may require surgical revision.

The pump reservoirs that hold the pain-relieving medication have to be filled monthly, requiring regular visits to the office of the physician who maintains the pump.

Successful spinal cord stimulation relieves 50 percent of pain in 75 percent of well-selected patients and still requires some additional pain-relieving medication. Spinal cord stimulators, though not implantable pumps, preclude the use of MRIs, particularly unfortunate in patients with spinal problems, who often need them to evaluate changes in their pain.

Leave the practice of any doctor who wants to implant one of these in you instead of giving you a reasonable narcotic regimen, such as six Percocet daily, possibly in combination with a long-acting drug such as MS Contin, Kadian, the Duragesic patch, or Oxycontin. (No preference is implied by the order of drugs listed.) Also, leave any doctor who says you need a high-tech implanted pain-relieving treatment because you are taking too much medication— even though that medication works and is well tolerated and you are not abusing it for addiction or psychological craving.

Get a Second Opinion

If a doctor tells you that you are not a candidate for a pain-relieving procedure, get a second opinion by one or two other physicians with recognized experience with it. If a physician tells you that a lesioning procedure theoretically could damage you, again consult with those who have significant practical experience performing it.

Some physicians who operate pain clinics are often trigger-happy with implantable devices: spinal-cord stimulators and pumps to deliver intraspinal medication. Many will tell you it is preferable to implant a device before contemplating the lesioning of nerves, especially performing a ganglion lesion. Rubbish. Radiofrequency lesions performed correctly are effective and safe. They help liberate you from the pain clinic: There is significant academic literature that proves it. They certainly liberate you more than an implantable device with its need for periodic maintenance.

Also, some limit the amount of oral or skin patch narcotics they supply, insisting that if you need more, you should try more epidurals or other interventions to relieve your pain. A strong economic incentive drives some of these postures.

Treatment of significant stenosis with epidurals is usually a waste of the patient's time and money and an exercise in wishful thinking for both patients and physicians who try it. The same applies to epidurals and root blocks for large disk herniations causing severe pain and weakness. Usually, by the time this kind of disk herniation heals on its own, most of us will be broke and depressed, on disability, or dead. Likewise, trying to control the severe back pain of someone with an unstable spine with epidurals, facet injections, disk procedures, and various radiofrequency lesions is just not going to work. The situations described above do not need interventional pain management; they need properly performed surgery. Obviously, there are patients who in the best of all worlds should undergo surgery but cannot for medical, psychological, or personal reasons. They must resign themselves to optimizing their existence, living their lives in some degree of chronic pain with ongoing medication and possibly a procedure from time to time.

For those who had surgery and still have significant postoperative pain, see the next chapter, on spinal surgery. The majority of patients with failed spine surgery require an accurate diagnosis and reoperation for insufficient decompression of their roots as a result of residual stenosis or disk fragments. If at all possible, people with residual root compression should not be treated with long-term pain management as a substitute for more definitive pain relief through properly performed decompressive surgery. For those with no anatomical basis for chronic postoperative pain, pain management is necessary.

Key Points to Choosing Interventional Treatments

- With treatment, always begin at the bottom of the ladder and work up. Start with the least invasive and conservative treatment, such as lifestyle changes and medications.
- Epidural steroid injections and some root blocks provide short-term relief of acute disk herniations and discogenic pain. Epidurals are often wrongly used instead of a trial of oral steroids.
- Nerve-root, facet, and branch blocks can temporarily relieve pain in damaged or compressed roots or painful facets but are best used as part of a diagnostic armamentarium to plan further, more definitive treatment.
- Radiofrequency lesioning can be used for long-term relief of pain in spinal structures supplied by nerves.
- Discogenic pain may be relieved by various procedures, including radiofrequency, IDET, and laser techniques.
- Vertebroplasty can be effective in treating pain from vertebrae that have acute osteoporotic fractures or metastatic tumors.
- Implantable devices, such as spinal stimulators and intraspinal drug delivery systems, can relieve pain not otherwise controllable.

Chapter 19

Treating Back Pain with Surgery

Spinal surgery, especially fusion, is vastly overused in this country. People often become tired of searching for a cure and agree to back surgery when it won't really do much good and may well marry them to future operations for the rest of their lives. On the other hand, spinal surgery is highly effective in certain conditions (when it should be performed earlier rather than later), such as a large disk herniation, significant spinal stenosis, cord compression resulting in signs of cord damage, and gross spinal instability with intractable pain that is attributable to that instability. When nerve damage is at risk, conservative therapy may not be enough.

Surgery is required if there is an ongoing disability from pain, weakness, difficulty walking, or signs of injury to the spinal cord. Surgery may be contemplated if you fail to improve with conservative therapy and also should be considered instead of conservative therapy for conditions that may result in permanent neurological injury. A conservative approach—bed rest and painkillers—must be tried for at least six to eight weeks before considering surgery. However, there are problems that require urgent surgical attention.

As a rule, the greater the dysfunction and the more quickly it appeared, the greater the urgency of surgery to avoid irreversible damage. A herniated disk in the neck or thoracic area that is causing arm or chest pain and is also pressing on the spinal cord and causing leg weakness, for example, should be surgically treated with haste. Weakness of the muscles that raise the foot off the ground or of those that keep your knee straight is a particularly troubling sign of a lower lumbar-disk herniation. If this weakness doesn't go away spontaneously or through surgery, you might end up with a permanent inability to walk normally.

Even without weakness or numbness, any ongoing disabling pain from disk herniation requires surgery if conservative therapy does not work. Just make sure that the herniation is clearly seen on a high-quality radiological study. Ask your doctor to show you the films of your spine. I always show them to my patients. It makes them feel better to see exactly what is going to happen during treatment. I also show them on a skeleton that I keep in my office. This is not a Halloween prop but a good tool to help patients understand how their spines work. If your spine doctor doesn't have a model skeleton in his or her office, I suggest you find another doctor.

LUMBAR DISCECTOMY

The most common spinal surgery is a lumbar discectomy, which is the removal of a herniated or ruptured disk that is pressing on nerves and causing symptoms. In the lumbar spine, the disk is approached from the easiest direction: the back; the nerve roots (cauda equina) are pushed safely aside. The nerve roots are more resistant to manipulation like this than the delicate spinal cord in the cervical and thoracic spine. (In these upper spinal areas, a discectomy is usually performed from the front of the body and must be accompanied by a fusion.) To gain access to the lumbar spinal canal for a discectomy, a small part of the bone overlying the herniated disk is removed to expose the nerve roots and the disk. This may be accompanied by a partial removal of the facet joint to widen either the spinal canal or a window through which the nerves leave the spine (foramen). From the back the surgeon can see the disk pressing on the front of the nerve roots and can carefully remove it, often in several pieces. Then the wound is closed.

Usually, a discectomy takes an hour in the operating room and requires a hospital stay of up to four days. It is usually performed under general anesthesia.

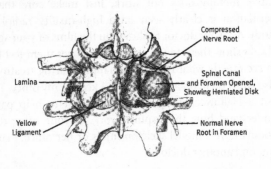

FIGURE 10. Rear view of lumbar spine, showing the right lamina and lower right facet extending from that lamina removed. A disk herniation is compressing a nerve root.

The day after surgery you can walk around the hospital room. Most people are well enough to go home by the fourth day and by six weeks can usually regain regular activity. The pain from the incision subsides gradually over several weeks. However, the weakened leathery disk covering (annulus) must be given time to heal. Heavy lifting, bending, and straining place increased pressure within the disk and strain the already weakened annulus. So avoid these activities for several months. If there is any level of slippage or instability at the level that was operated on, take it easy longer. Making the spine more unstable may result in the need for a fusion.

Your work and lifestyle influence your ability to return to work as much as anything else. A writer working at home can begin to work in the first few days after surgery; a plumber or athlete would put himself at risk by returning too soon.

If you are elderly, you may need rehabilitation for reconditioning more than for pain relief. Younger patients in general don't need rehab.

Once the compression is removed, the pain from the nerve root is significantly relieved, but it may linger for a few weeks, sometimes months. Weakness and numbness also diminish quickly. The duration and severity of the preoperative pain, weakness, and numbness influences the speed and extent of full recovery. Some people may have permanent residual pain; others may have some permanent weakness or numbness even if the pain disappears.

Chronic problems may exist after disk surgery. Pain or preoperative dysfunction may persist or a new, different pain, and new dysfunction may appear after surgery. This usually means one or more of the following: not all of the disk that compressed the root was removed at surgery, the root was damaged by the disk pressing on it before surgery, the spine slipped or there was more disk herniation just after surgery, or the root was damaged in the attempt to remove the disk.

If new neurological dysfunction occurs after surgery, a thorough reevaluation with an MRI and usually a CT/myelogram with flexion-extension views is needed. You may want to get a second or third opinion on what appears to have been a failed operation. In the long run, you may require another operation or permanent chronic pain management.

In general, surgery makes an intolerable condition tolerable. Sixty-five percent to 80 percent of discectomy patients have no leg pain a year after surgery compared with 36 percent of patients who declined surgery. Most of us cannot wait for months for the expected resolution of a disk herniation. Surgical treatment of radicular symptoms from disk herniations is safe and cost-effective.

Open Surgery

Open lumbar disk surgery is 85 percent to 95 percent successful. At a minimum of five years after surgery, 62 percent of people in one study had complete relief of back and leg pain, 96 percent were pleased that they underwent surgery.

There is approximately a 1 percent rate of serious complications with open discectomy. These include infections of the surgical wound or the disk remaining in the spine (remember, only the piece of disk pressing on the nerves is removed, not the whole disk). These require antibiotics and possibly more surgery.

Another complication is a tear in the dura, the otherwise watertight covering that encases the cord and cauda, causing leakage of spinal fluid into the surgical wound. This tear has to be repaired. If the tear is not recognized and is sutured closed at the time of surgery, more surgery to close it may be required in a few days.

Damage to the nerves can occur, resulting in temporary or permanent weakness, numbness, pain, or bowel, bladder, or sexual dysfunction. The rate of death from this kind of surgery is less than one in a hundred, even for people over seventy-five.

Microdiscectomy

Microdiscectomy is a thirty-year-old procedure that is performed using an operating microscope. It uses a smaller incision and hole in the spine to remove the herniated disk. It is not clear whether there is a better outcome with this than with standard disk-removal surgery. However, the surgeon can charge a higher fee for using the operating microscope, even briefly, during surgery. A microdiscectomy may have a higher failure rate than the traditional discectomy because the herniated disk material may not always be seen and therefore removed as completely as in surgery through a slightly larger opening in the spinal canal. Surgery must therefore be repeated to finish the job.

Percutaneous Discectomy

Percutaneous discectomy, which is performed by pushing instruments through the skin without an incision, sounds great. However, it doesn't work as well as open surgical procedures. Like microdiscectomy, this incisionless procedure has a higher failure rate than traditional discectomy and a greater need for reoperation. I don't believe the percutaneous procedure can reliably solve the problems caused by many disk herniations.

Emergency Surgery for Disk Herniation

Emergency surgery is needed when a large piece of disk is herniated suddenly into the spinal canal causing severe weakness and numbness in the arms and legs, or bowel and bladder dysfunction. Such symptoms can also be caused by a broken vertebra, tumor, infection, or blood clot and must be treated urgently.

The longer the neural structures—especially the spinal cord—are compressed, the less likely is recovery. If the pressure is not quickly taken off the nerves or cord, strength, sensation, and bodily functions can be impaired. In addition to the neurological dysfunction mentioned, it may also cause severe burning, throbbing, and aching pain forever. This creates a need for constant pain medication, perhaps even the use of implantable devices to control the pain (see Chapters 17 and 18).

Disk-Replacement Surgery

Avoid this surgery. Medical science has now made it possible to replace degenerating disks just as is done with knees and hips. However, replacement parts wear out; in five to ten years you may need another operation replacing that disk with a new one. Moreover, the operation to accomplish the removal and replacement is much more invasive than a simple discectomy; it usually requires an incision into the abdomen or flank. This is a very controversial experimental procedure, not widely used. We have no long-term studies to show how effective—or ineffective—it is.

FORAMENOTOMY

This elegant, minimalist surgery is underutilized by many spine surgeons, especially in the cervical and thoracic areas. This procedure is used to relieve compression of nerve roots from disk herniation or arthritic narrowing.

In a foramenotomy the surgeon approaches the foramen—the bony hole or window through which a root leaves the spine—from the back and partially (in the lumbar spine) or completely (in the cervical and thoracic spine) drills off the back of the window. Once the pressure on the nerve root has been removed, the pain and dysfunction from the disk herniation or stenosis subsides, even if the disk in front of the root is left intact. Disks in or near the foramen in the lumbar spine may be removed (discectomy), though only with some difficulty, if they are new and not calcified. If they are calcified, a foramenotomy is performed, and they are left in place. In the neck, disks in the foramen are usually left in place and treated with a foramenotomy or, less elegantly, a fusion from the front of the neck. Cervical foramen narrowed by arthritic overgrowth may be treated with good success with a foramenotomy. Similarly, in the thoracic spine, a foramenotomy is usually performed to open the foramen when a calcified ligament or a herniated disk compresses the root. In a recent study of thoracic disks that caused chronic pain by pressing on nerve roots exiting the spine, 84 percent of patients who underwent surgery from the back (the foramenotomy type of surgery) had good to excellent results. The time in the operating room and hospital is similar to that for a discectomy. The demands of your work and lifestyle also influence recovery time.

If you have a disk herniation or narrowing of the foramen from arthritis, seek out a surgeon with expertise in this technique. In the right person, foramenotomies may be performed with excellent results, permitting the avoidance of far more complicated fusion surgery in the neck and thoracic spine.

LAMINOTOMY, LAMINECTOMY, AND PARTIAL FACETECTOMY FOR LUMBAR STENOSIS

These are all terms describing surgical procedures for taking pressure off nerve roots.

- Laminotomy is the removal of a portion of the lamina, the bony arches of the vertebrae that cover the back of the spinal canal and the nerve roots. Hemilaminotomy is the partial removal of the

     lamina on either side. Bilateral hemilaminotomy
     is partial removal of the lamina on both sides.
- Laminectomy is the complete removal of the
   entire lamina: the back of the entire canal.
   Hemilaminectomy is the complete removal
   of the lamina on either side.
- Partial facetectomy is the partial removal of the
   facet joint. Indeed, the inner or medial third of
   the joint usually is removed (medial facetectomy).
- The usual surgical treatment for lumbar stenosis
   is laminotomy or laminectomy and facetectomy.

Surgery for stenosis should always include a medial facetectomy, which is shaving off the inner third of the facet and
opening the spinal canal to make more room for the nerve
roots on the side of the canal. When it is properly performed,
this surgery has excellent results. Often the foramen may
need further opening (foramenotomy), as it may have
become tightened by arthritic overgrowth that presses the
nerve roots coursing through it.

    It takes about an hour at each lumbar level to perform
this surgery. Stenosis surgery may be done at only one level
or as many as five. Patients usually leave the hospital in four
days and recover from their postoperative pain in a few
weeks. Many need no rehabilitation after surgery and gradually resume normal activity over the next six weeks to a few
months. People who had put off the surgery for a long time
and became unable to take more than a few steps around the
house may need two weeks of inpatient rehabilitation and a
few weeks of physical therapy on their own.

    This is a good operation for the elderly. Approximately 65
percent of patients have good results from this type of surgery for stenosis. When they don't do well with stenosis sur-

gery in the low back, it is often because they had an insignificant removal of the inner third of the facets or opening of
the foramen, or it may be that they have so many spinal
problems that it is impossible to safely address all of them
this way.

Thirty percent to 40 percent of those who have the operation do not get long-lasting benefit. However, remember
that stenosis is usually a condition of diffusely aging spines,
often with disk degeneration and arthritic abnormalities at
multiple levels. The most severe problem—the one causing
the present symptoms—may be corrected in one operation
with excellent results. However, the aging process and spinal
degeneration will continue. In a few years, another level may
begin to cause problems and eventually require surgical
treatment. Surgery is not a cure for the aging process, but for
the pain of severe stenosis, which limits the ability to walk,
surgery can give gratifying results.

SPINAL FUSION: APPROACH WITH CAUTION

A fusion is an operation in which one or more vertebrae
of the spine are fused together with another piece of bone
(your own or, more rarely, a sterile piece from a cadaver
bone bank), often with the help of an attachment of rigid
metal hardware to the operated-on area of the spine.

If your own bone is used, it is usually taken from the
inside or back of your pelvis. There will be some pain in that
area for a few days after surgery. In a few patients, it may be
long-lasting. Not all fusions successfully fuse the vertebrae
together. Fusions with your own bone are more likely to take
and are less costly than those done with bone purchased
from a cadaver bone bank. Using your own bone is sometimes impossible though, especially in large operations for
spinal tumors in which the vertebrae are removed, replaced

with large pieces of bank bone, and fused with hardware. The bone laid down for the fusion is often in the form of small blocks, and it takes time—six to eight weeks in the neck, three months in the thoracic-lumbar area—for the blocks to grow together to form a solid union. The metallic hardware is to hold the spine stable until the bony fusion takes hold. After that, it stays in place. It has no real purpose thereafter except in patients with major scoliosis surgery where it helps support the spine.

Fusion of any kind requires more time in the operating room than the other operations mentioned. A one-level cervical fusion takes about an hour and a quarter, certainly less than two hours. It is usually performed with a bone graft without hardware. Hardware may be used if the surgery involves multiple levels. However, the surgeon, the number of levels fused, the nature of the patient's problem, and even his lifestyle also play a role in formulating the technical aspects of the operation. Fusing one lumbar level (L_{4-5}) from the back or through the abdomen using hardware takes two to two and a half hours. Thoracic fusions are performed with hardware and usually take several hours whether they are done from the back or front. The more extensive the fusion at any level of the spine and the more hardware it takes, the more time it takes. Complex lumbar fusions or scoliosis surgery may take four to eleven hours. Sometimes several operations are needed. A complex fusion may be performed first from the back then, usually a few days later, from the front.

Recovery from a fusion is more painful and longer than other back surgery. It can take four to five months for a major scoliosis operation. For the right patient in the long run it is well worth it. To recover from fusion surgery, it is important to resume activity only in a slowly progressive fashion. This allows you to regain power and mobility as the fusion heals and prevent painful spinal instability.

Any spinal fusion—in the neck, thoracic area, or lower back—distorts the normal movement of your spine. The segments above and below the fused area move excessively, compensating for the lack of movement in the fused segment. The excessive movement accelerates wear. Disks herniate, stenosis from arthritic buildup occurs, even instability can occur; problems that must be addressed in the five to ten years following fusion, often by more surgery, possibly even further fusion. At least 10 percent of patients require more surgery following thoracic-lumbar fusions and I suspect a similar statistic applies to cervical fusions. At least 30 percent of people who undergo thoracic-lumbar fusion later have serious complications. These include severe low back pain and increased spinal degeneration above and below the fusion. Thirty percent to 70 percent of patients who undergo thoracic-lumbar fusions never return to work. It is not always clear why some patients with fusions have significant chronic pain. Assuming a fusion was successful, some surgeons blame the hardware for chronic postoperative pain. Unfortunately, I have rarely seen chronic pain following lumbar fusion improve following removal of the allegedly offending hardware.

The United States is in the midst of an epidemic of lumbar fusions not unlike the epidemic of hysterectomies and cesareans of a few years ago. From 1995 to 1996, neck and thoracic fusion each increased close to threefold and lumbar fusion increased by 21 percent. Neck fusion is the biggest category in fusion surgery (48 percent), followed by lumbar (33 percent), and thoracic (13 percent). Our nation has by far the highest incidence of spinal surgery in the world. The rate of fusion varies by region. The Midwest and South do more than the Northeast, which in turn does more than the West. This is not because an Alabama back differs from a Boston back but because of the biases and experience or lack of it of physicians.

Even more striking is the tremendous variability of the rate of fusion within one area. It is tenfold between communities within a hundred-mile radius in northern New England, and there is a sixfold variation between two surgeons in the same hospital. There may be other reasons for this epidemic of fusion. Several studies concluded that both doctors and hospitals obtain more revenue from fusion than from simpler operations.

There is no data that suggests fusion is better than simple laminectomy for treating disk herniations or uncomplicated spinal stenosis. Nor is there any data that suggests fusion is any better than any other therapy in treating pain from sore but not herniated disks: discogenic pain, usually defined by a discogram. Yet as of 1998, 51 percent of lumbar fusions were performed for disk-related pain, 11 percent for stenosis. Many more fusions—especially for patients with stenosis—are performed each year, many seemingly unnecessary. The bottom line: have a fusion only if you must and by the surgeon with the most experience with this surgery that you can find.

When Fusion Is Appropriate

A spinal fusion should be done only when pain cannot be relieved by other means or if there is significant weakness, numbness, or bowel or bladder problems and appropriate X-rays reveal ongoing slippage—abnormal movement—between adjoining vertebrae that explains the problems.

There are situations where fusion is appropriate. First, to remove a herniated disk in the neck or thoracic spine that is pressing on the spinal cord or nerves. Remember, the disks lie between the vertebral bodies in front of the cord or in the lumbar spine, the cauda equina. In the cervical and thoracic spine, a discectomy is best approached from the front, entering the spine through the disk space of the offending disk and proceeding from the front to the back of the disk and surrounding vertebra. The cord is least likely to be damaged this way. Once the disk is removed, a fusion must be undertaken to restore spinal stability.

Fusion may be necessary to correct the deformity and side effects of scoliosis, reconstruct the spine in patients who have tumors of the spine or whose spine has been broken in an accident.

Another reason for fusion is instability of the spine—the bones slipping one over another—that causes intractable pain with or without weakness or numbness.

Neck (Cervical) Fusion

Fusions from the front of the neck are regularly performed today with good results. They require less than a week of hospital stay and a three-month recovery. More than 87 percent of patients who undergo fusion of the neck from the front have good-to-excellent results. The rate of failed fusion increases with the number of spinal levels fused. In the cervical spine, the need for reoperation occurs in one in five fusions.

Fusions from the front of the neck may be performed by using a piece of bone inserted into the surgical cavity in the disk space and between the vertebral bodies. Fusions from the front of the neck may or may not involve hardware, depending on various factors noted above. Fusion in the neck may be performed from the back of the neck as well, usually to stabilize a spine that has slipped because of trauma or tumors. These fusions always use metallic wires or other hardware.

Lumbar Fusion

Fusion should not be done in the lower back unless the spine slips back and forth and continues to do so and you have disabling, poorly controlled pain or weakness, significant numbness, or another neurological problem. Even if your spine slips, if you can find a way to live with it, do not have a fusion because the fusion itself can cause chronic pain. There are some things about the biomechanics of the fused spine that we have not yet begun to understand.

Thoracic Fusion

Thoracic fusions can correct scoliosis, including cerebral palsy, polio, or other neurological diseases. It is also used to treat spinal damage from trauma (broken vertebrae), infections, and tumors. Thoracic disk herniations are often treated with this technique as well.

In thoracic fusion, the surgeon approaches the spine through either the front of the thorax (chest cavity), the back of the spine, or both. Fusion from the front of the chest starts with an incision under the ribs. Because the pressure of bending the thoracic spine creates the possibility of breakdown of thoracic fusion with subsequent damage to the underlying spinal cord, metallic hardware is used to fix the fusion.

Thoracic fusion is big surgery requiring a potentially long, painful recovery and should only be undertaken if it is absolutely necessary. When needed, this kind of fusion corrects deformities, arrests progressive deformity, corrects breathing problems from deformity, removes pressure on nerve roots and the spinal cord, and to some extent, relieves pain.

Why Fusions Fail

Not all fusions take. The vertebrae do not always become fused together by the blocks of bone laid down during surgery. It is important for you to know that fusions don't always work. In assuring the success of any fusion, it is important to let the bones fuse by avoiding excessive activity in the weeks and even months following surgery. Smoking and the use of some nonsteroidal painkillers may interfere with fusion. In such cases, another operation with another fusion may be needed. In addition to the type of bone used (see above), and the extent of a fusion is also related to failure. In the neck, the rate of failed fusion increases with the number of levels fused, from negligible to about 10 percent for single level and as high as 27 percent for two or more levels. However, in the cervical spine, the need for another operation because of pain or other problems occurs in only up to one in six failed fusion patients.

In an analysis of twenty studies of lumbar fusions, the average failure rate was 14 percent and varied according to the technique used. If the original failed fusion was performed from the back, as is common, the second corrective fusion will usually be made through the abdomen. This is much bigger surgery than fusion from the back.

To maximize the chances of success of fusion, you should have it performed by a highly experienced surgeon. You also need to give the bones the best chance to fuse by being cautious about activity after surgery, not smoking before or after surgery, and using NSAIDs or other pain relievers after surgery to ease pain.

COMPLICATIONS OF BACK SURGERY

Everyone who undergoes spinal surgery in which the inside of the spine is invaded—as in disk surgery—develops some scarring. The majority recover without developing chronic pain. Chronic postoperative pain in many people indicates inadequate surgery, that something is still pressing on the nerve roots, or spinal instability was unrecognized before surgery. However, it can also be caused by the operation itself: trauma to the nerves. Traumatized nerves are usually inflamed and may develop scars within them. This may result in numbness or an abnormal sensation of the skin supplied by them, weakness, and aching, burning, or tingling pain. Surgery to remove scars of any kind inside the spine is usually not only unsuccessful but often causes even more damage than there was before. If a surgeon suggests treating your chronic postoperative pain with another operation to remove the scar tissue, find another surgeon. The same thing applies to the use of as yet unproven pain-management techniques to relieve epidural scars—epiduroscopy (an invasive technique to see into the epidural space) and injections of chemicals.

Failed back surgery syndrome (FBSS) is the persistence or the onset of low back pain or leg pain after spinal surgery. It is estimated that 66 percent of patients in pain clinics suffer from this problem. There are various causes: they include inadequate stenosis surgery, recurrent disk herniation, and residual disk fragments. Persistent neck or arm pain after neck surgery is less common, and since neck surgery is several times less common than lumbar surgery, failed neck surgery syndrome plays a small role in most pain clinics. (This is not a contradiction to what was stated above. Cervical fusions are indeed more common than lumbar fusions, but there is more to spine surgery than fusions.) Persistent thoracic pain after thoracic surgery— usually fusions—can certainly occur, but fewer patients have this problem after surgery than have chronic neck pain. People with residual pain problems after surgery shouldn't necessarily receive long-term pain management but should be given the opportunity for prolonged relief through another, correctly performed, operation if needed.

If after surgery you continue to suffer from pain, either you still have nerve root compression, your roots or cord was damaged by the compression before surgery or was damaged in the surgery, or you may be one of a large number of patients with otherwise successful lumbar or thoracic fusions who continue to experience back and even leg pain.

The source of chronic postoperative pain has to be determined by a complete reevaluation with a careful history, examination, possible electrodiagnostic studies, and high-quality radiological studies, including, in many cases, a CT/myelogram with flexion/extension views. This reevaluation should be performed by your surgeon or a neurologist with special competence and interest in spinal problems. A second or third opinion may be sought if you are told that the operation went well and that there is no anatomical basis for your pain. Do not accept the comment that "your surgery went well and you should not have chronic pain" unless a competent postoperative evaluation has been diligently conducted.

A delightful young nurse practitioner suffered a horrible surgical mishap while undergoing what was a probably unnecessary lumbar fusion. One of the surgeons placed a screw to hold the fusion together through a nerve going down into her right leg. He removed the screw in the operating room, but the damage was done. She awoke with severe right leg pain and required a catheter to urinate. Her foot and part of her leg and the right half of her vagina and rectum were numb. She also developed severe low-back pain. She had not worked at all for four months when she saw me and was seriously thinking of declaring permanent disability. She was taking some minor painkillers and nonanalgesic antidepressants in a disorganized fashion with no apparent relief of pain or depression.

She consulted me for control of her pain and an explanation of what had happened. (No one had really explained it to her.) After obtaining a series of radiological studies, I understood the damage done by the screw. I told her that she would need some form of pain medication for the rest of her life. I also told her I wanted to try to help her return to work if she and her former employer would work with me.

Over the next two months we fine-tuned a complicated drug regimen to control most of the side effects well enough for her to work. Her nerve injury had damaged some of the nerves used for bowel and bladder function. A urologist was able, with some new medication, to help her void better. We effectively combated her residual sleepiness with Ritalin, an amphetamine. After she had been living for a while on her new drug regimen, she shed tears of joy because something had finally been done to help her.

I am pleased that with a reasonable amount of pain relief, psychotherapy, and medication for depression, she went back to work as a nurse practitioner three days a week and enjoys the challenge of her job. She obviously still carries a lot of physical and psychological baggage around with her, but she is stronger now and can carry it more easily. These results are not exceptional. I had simply done my job, the task of any physician who treats pain.

DOCTORS WHO PERFORM SPINAL SURGERY

Not all neurosurgeons specialize in spinal surgery. Don't see a neurosurgeon for a spinal problem unless he or she has a particularly good reputation in whatever you need done: disk or stenosis surgery or possible spinal fusion. Thoracic spinal surgery is less common than surgery in the lumbar spine or neck, so if you have a thoracic disk herniation, don't go to your local neurosurgeron if he or she has performed only two thoracic disk operations. Some excellent neurosurgeons with great expertise in treating spinal problems do not perform low-back and thoracic fusions without the help of another surgeon skilled in them. Orthopedic spinal surgeons are best able to treat scoliosis.

Orthopedic surgeons are more likely to suggest fusion than many neurosurgeons. If a surgeon says you need a fusion, find one or, better yet, two neurosurgeons or orthopedists who are conservative about it. If they say you need one, you probably do.

The more complicated the surgery, the more research you should do and the more opinions you should get. If you talk to a doctor about surgery, be sure to ask these questions or have these demonstrations of your condition:

- What is wrong with me?
- Show me what is wrong on my radiological studies. (Seeing the actual film will help you understand what is wrong with your back.)
- Show me on a skeleton what is wrong with my back.
- If I am not a candidate for surgery, what should I do?
- If I am a candidate for surgery but wish to delay it or refuse to have it, what can I do?
- If I am a candidate for surgery, what surgical treatments do you suggest for my condition?
- Do I really need a fusion, or can I get by quite well with a simpler operation, like a simple discectomy or foramenotomy?
- What are the upsides and downsides of surgery?
- What is the recovery like?
- How many of these surgeries have you performed?
- If you are not a spine surgeon, what surgeons do you recommend and why?

- Can I speak to a patient who had a good outcome from the operation you propose?
- Can I speak to someone who did not fare as well with the proposed surgery?

Key Points about Spinal Surgery

- Spinal surgery, especially fusion, is vastly overused in this country.
- Surgery is needed if there is an ongoing disability from pain, weakness, or bowel or bladder dysfunction.
- The most common spinal surgery is a lumbar discectomy to remove herniated disk pressing on nerves.
- Avoid disk replacement surgery until long-term studies have proven it safe and effective.
- Emergency spinal surgery is needed to rapidly decompress a spinal cord or nerve roots under sudden pressure and causing a significant dysfunction such as weakness, numbness, or loss of body function.
- Always get more than one opinion before you agree to spinal surgery.
- Always ask to see the films of your spine and have the problem explained on the films and a skeleton.

Chapter 20

Eastern Needling and Other Integrative Means of Pain Relief

Many alternative or complementary therapies can make you feel good, but they will not necessarily cure your back pain unless they are used with traditional medical care or as part of an integrated treatment program. People come to alternative or complementary therapy for a variety of reasons, including a friend's recommendation or a television advertisement.

If Western medicine had all the answers, no other therapy would be sought. The term complementary medicine implies that these therapies are to be used in concert with conventional therapies for pain. The term alternative therapy suggests that these therapies are mutually exclusive. However, this is not always true. All therapy should be scientifically evaluated. Ineffective treatment of any kind should be abandoned.

Americans spend $27 billion a year on herbal remedies, chiropractors, and massage therapists. In the 1990s, as the popularity of alternative medicine grew and the cost of traditional medicine soared, the National Institutes of Health began to fund studies that would provide the public with useful information on the effectiveness of treatment other than the traditional. In 1998 the *Journal of the American Medical Association* published studies identifying some nontraditional treatments that seemed to work and others that were ineffective. However, we still don't know very much about their long-term effects.

Throughout human history, we have used healing techniques we now call complementary therapy. Some of these therapies were developed in India and China well before modern scientific methods developed. For some of them, we still do not know the exact mechanism of action. Some physicians believe that the benefits are largely from the placebo effect, that is, that the act of doing the therapy rather than the therapy itself makes you feel better. Nevertheless, more attention is now paid to nontraditional medicine in medical schools and by practicing physicians, some of whom have actually learned how to give acupuncture treatments.

Always tell your doctor about every vitamin, herbal supplement, exercise, or manual therapy you use. He or she may have experience with complementary practitioners and be able to offer recommendations. These therapies are here to stay, and some may help your back pain, at least temporarily.

Use them wisely to:

- ease symptoms of chronic pain, stress, and anxiety
- enhance the effects of conventional medical treatment
- improve your overall mood and outlook

In general, complementary therapies cannot replace conventional therapy, cure an illness, or quickly improve an acute condition. The potential for harm from some alternative therapy, such as herbal remedies, is often a result of patients who use alternative medicine without telling their physicians that they are doing so. For example, the herb Saint-John's-wort may result in serious complications during anesthesia for surgery. The anesthesiologist needs to avoid some drugs in patients using this herb or serious harm may result. Aside from this, if my patients find that alternative medicine and therapies work for them, I am happy for them as long as there are no untoward side effects from the treatment.

In the long run, the role of acupuncture and other traditional or nontraditional pain-control methods has to be determined through outcome studies.

Ask these questions before you undertake any therapy:

- How effective is the treatment and for how long?
- What are the costs and risks?
- How does it compare with other treatments for the same problem?
- May I see your license and credentials?

ACUPUNCTURE

Acupuncture is an ancient Chinese therapeutic process in which specific points of the body are stimulated with needles to foster healing or pain relief. The theory is that the body's energy—chi—is carried along pathways, called meridians. When you are ill, the flow of chi in the twelve primary meridians is out of synch. If specific points along the meridians are stimulated the flow can be corrected to optimize health or block pain. Western researchers theorize that where acupuncture eases pain, it does so by stimulating the central nervous system to release chemicals (endorphins) that lessen the perception of pain.

Thin needles are used for the 360 specific points along the meridians. As few as five or as many as fifteen sterile needles are inserted from a mere fraction of an inch to four inches deep. As the needles are inserted, you may feel a light needle prick or tingling, warmth, or pinching. The needles are left in place from five to sixty minutes. Twenty minutes is about the average. A course of ten treatments is usually needed to obtain maximum benefit. Follow-up treatments, usually every few months, are advised to maintain normal energy balance. Some therapists may use heat, pressure, friction, suction, or electrical current in addition to needles or in place of them.

However it works, acupuncture has a role in the management of short-term acute pain and seems to have some benefit for the treatment of some chronic pain syndromes, such as shoulder aches from arthritis, joint aches, and muscle strain. There is no evidence yet that acupuncture is effective in treating chronic back pain. Theoretically, acupuncture might relieve significant spinal pain of various origins—disk herniations, arthritis, stenosis, and muscular, for example— for at least a short time, just as it has been used to control pain during surgery in China. That won't make much of a dent on even a two-week course of leg pain (radiculopathy) from a disk herniation, much less chronic spinal pain as is typical in arthritis and stenosis. Maybe a severe bout of myofascial or diffuse muscle spasm pain can be reversed through acupuncture.

The United States Food and Drug Administration estimates that 9 to 12 million patients spend as much as $500 million on acupuncture treatments each year. In the year 2000, an estimated twenty thousand licensed acupuncturists were practicing in thirty-four states and the District of Columbia. In 1999, more than three thousand medical doctors trained in acupuncture practiced; there was at least one in every state.

Does It Help Low-Back Pain?

I have sent some patients with musculoskeletal pain to acupuncturists, usually after they have asked me about the treatment. It was evident, however, that few found sustained relief. My own observations are echoed in a medical report in *Spine* a few years ago that surveyed various studies on the effect of acupuncture on low-back pain. The results were decidedly negative. Of eleven studies, only two were of high scientific quality. They showed no benefit to acupuncture over such treatments as TENS (see Chapter 16). But because it is important to exhaust all forms of treatment before progressing to more costly and serious interventions and since at least a modest percentage of patients with chronic lumbar spine pain from arthritis or trauma improved somewhat during a course of acupuncture treatment, this alternative deserves our attention.

Possible Risks

So far we do not have good data on the frequency of a positive response to acupuncture treatments. Acupuncture is something to consider if toxic side effects prevent the use of medications. However, it is a passive, time-consuming procedure that is also relatively expensive (and is not yet universally covered by medical insurance).

Acupuncture has a good safety record when it's done by a licensed practitioner. However, there are possible complications, such as infections (AIDS or hepatitis), if nonsterile needles are used. The therapist should use sterile disposable needles so that there is no chance of infection. Theoretically, organs may be punctured; and local bleeding may occur, causing a large bruise, especially in patients on blood thinners such as aspirin or other NSAIDs or, worse, Coumadin.

MANUAL MANIPULATION

Chiropractors, osteopaths, and massage therapists believe that the body's natural healing processes are facilitated through the manipulation and movement of soft tissues and the repositioning of body parts. They claim that their treatment removes blockages and results in improved function; that they move the spine back to its normal position. These manipulators are also very popular with people who cannot get relief from back pain from their medical doctors.

Chiropractic manipulation has been the subject of studies and stories that offer a conflicting picture as to whether such treatment is beneficial. Responding to this situation and aware of the popularity of chiropractics, the National Institutes of Health has funded studies to look into its effectiveness. Scant published research indicates that physical manipulation of sore tight body parts does make people feel better. My own opinion is a guarded one, especially when it is treatment for head, neck, and shoulder pain.

Chiropractors have caused strokes by twisting the neck in such a way that arteries that pass through holes in the vertebrae of the upper spine to the brain become kinked, thus closing off a blood vessel. Inadequate blood supply to the brain from a kinked vessel can result in permanent nerve damage, even in the young. A few years ago I treated a woman of twenty-seven who had suffered a stroke at the base of her brain; it was induced by her chiropractor. She had risk factors for the stroke: She was taking birth control pills, smoked, was taking decongestants, and had used cocaine shortly before the manipulation. She was under the care of a doctor who prescribed strong decongestants for chronic sinusitis. She went to the chiropractor for control of her neck pain. As soon as the chiropractor pulled her neck, she felt weakness and numbness in the face and part of one side of her body. She ultimately recovered, returned to work, married, and had children. Only a patch of residual numbness in her face persisted.

Vigorous manipulation of the neck may damage the spinal cord of anyone with spinal-cord compression from a disk, arthritic overgrowth, or a tumor. Spinal cord damage can result in permanent nerve damage, including paralysis. Manipulating an unstable spine can be disastrous: it may damage the fragile spinal cord within the bony spine. Chiropractors and massage therapists often do not obtain MRIs and other sophisticated radiological studies that can guide diagnosis and treatment. Chiropractors usually do obtain simple X-rays of the spine, which can alert them to the presence of a grossly unstable spine, which they should not manipulate.

The Laying on of Hands

One reason chiropractic manipulation makes people feel better is that they are being therapeutically touched. According to a study of 321 adults with only low-back pain (without sciatica), reading a booklet about back pain (and having no treatment) was about as effective as chiropractic manipulation or physical therapy in treating low-back pain. However, 70 percent of the participants who had experienced the two physically oriented therapies were happy with their treatment versus only 30 percent of those who had done nothing but read the booklet. Reading is far less expensive and more convenient than visiting an office; however, people would rather have someone listen to them and be physically touched by a health professional. "Laying on of hands" is an intrinsic part of the healing process, something that is missing in today's health-care system.

The differences between the types of manipulation performed by osteopaths and chiropractors and some massage therapists may not be striking; they depend on the practitioner and the patient being treated. A 1999 study lends some support to the use of osteopathic manipulation to treat low-back pain. In patients with low-back pain, this kind of manipulation was demonstrated to be equally effective as standard medical care, such as muscle relaxants, analgesics, NSAIDS, physical therapy, and TENS. Whether they received osteopathic or standard medical treatment, patients were equally pleased with their care and accepted their back problem well. However, those treated by standard care were likely to spend more on medication and physical therapy, resulting in higher treatment costs. This study thus provides an economic argument for using spinal manipulation in treating some kinds of low-back pain, such as that caused by muscle spasm.

Osteopaths and chiropractors are trained differently. Unlike chiropractors, osteopaths receive a degree (DO or Doctor of Osteopathy) that is the equivalent to a medical degree, except that they also learn a form of spinal manipulation in their training that physicians with MDs do not.

Spending time and money on spinal manipulation or physical therapy twice a week for long periods of time is usually not the best way to deal with chronic pain if there are more effective or less time-consuming therapies available.

Therapeutic Massage

Hippocrates, the father of medicine, believed that massage freed nutritive fluids to flow to the body's organs. The

Romans took this a step further and made massage part of their healing system. Eastern cultures in India and China also developed massage techniques, and today we have various massage styles. In today's fast-paced, largely sedentary world, spas that offer massage have become increasingly popular for stress relief.

Western massage, such as Swedish, is designed to relax tense muscles to improve range of motion, remove stress, and increase energy. Putting pressure on muscles brings a different sensation into the tissues and relieves pain. Chinese and Japanese forms of massage, such as shiatsu, improve the flow of energy—chi—through the body's energy channels. Pressure on acupuncture points releases blocked chi and restores the body's natural balance.

Work with a licensed massage therapist (LMT) who uses therapeutic muscle massage to improve musculoskeletal disorders rather than someone with no medical training who was hired by the health club or spa. Massage techniques vary from a light touch to a more vigorous stretching of muscles. Some use a lot of pummeling and poking and can often cause you to tense up because it hurts. Ask what kind of technique you will get beforehand. Explain what you are looking for.

Experienced masseurs deliver the best sessions, so find a practitioner who knows the particulars of your back condition. Contact organizations that certify massage therapists or your state's licensing board to check the status of the practitioner you are considering. Gather recommendations from other health professionals or the practitioner's patients. Massage can relieve muscular pain, whether it be primary or secondary to an underlying disk herniation. It cannot relieve the pain emanating from deeper structures: disk herniations or annular tears, chronically painful facets, stenosis, spinal instability, or tumors.

MIND-BODY THERAPIES

Pain is heightened by negative emotions and anxiety, which increase muscle tension and may lead to depression. Improving your emotional state will have a beneficial effect on your physical status. Mind-body therapies include biofeedback, hypnosis, relaxation techniques, and meditation. They may increase your sense of self-control and accomplishment, but they don't all work for everyone. Investigate the technique that appeals to you; if one doesn't help, try another. Mind-body therapies require time and effort, but they have few side effects and are inexpensive.

Relaxation

In his book, *The Relaxation Response,* Dr. Herbert Benson popularized a technique that has been successfully used to treat various kinds of pain, including back pain. The response is often subjectively experienced as a sense of well-being, peace of mind, and feeling at ease with the world. All of these constitute an altered state of consciousness, which slows down your breathing, lowers blood pressure, relaxes muscles, and changes your brain-wave activity. This response is the opposite of the fight-or-flight response to fear or an emergency situation, including pain. There are a variety of techniques to reach this state, but you need to relax. Repetition of a word or sound, known as a mantra, often helps. Transcendental meditation is one technique for achieving this response.

An important feature of this relaxation response is its prolonged benefit, which far outlasts the actual relaxing mental exercise. It appears that pain is perceived differently under the influence of this response. Pain impulses are still transmitted (body) but are perceived with less suffering (mind). It is as if the alarm reaction of the mind is somehow deconditioned and no longer responds with the same magnitude when confronted by bodily pain. The relaxation response can give you some relief and a sense of mastery over your condition.

There are a variety of ways to produce the relaxation response. Deep-breathing exercises may calm the sympathetic nervous system (it controls some of your vital functions, such as heart rate and blood pressure), thereby reducing pulse and blood pressure and, more important, relaxing tight muscles. If you are relaxed, you are likely to experience less pain than if you are anxious or depressed. Once you learn how to breathe deeply from the abdomen, you can get into a relaxed state at any time. Place your hand over your abdomen as it rises when you inhale and deflates when you exhale. Keep breathing slowly. If you breathe too rapidly, you may become dizzy and develop muscle cramps. This simple breathing exercise and other relaxation techniques can be used to reduce the intensity of the pain.

There are many books available for such relaxation techniques as progressive muscle relaxation, a technique that contracts muscles then relaxes them, beginning with the feet and moving up through the body.

Relaxation techniques are free of side effects and cost nothing. They do require lots of effort on your part to gain the benefit.

Meditation

Meditation reduces tension and helps relieve pain. You need a quiet place without distractions to meditate and a sitting posture that is comfortable and stable (the crossed-legged lotus position is not necessary). Meditation begins with deep breathing focusing thoughts on a meaningful word, phrase, or object. Over time, silent repetition of a word, such as "om," or a phrase changes your consciousness. Your mind will wander and chatter; the trick is to stick with the practice long enough to relax and improve concentration.

Hypnosis

Hypnosis or even self-hypnosis may help alleviate painful conditions in some people. It has been successfully used with cancer pain, in dentistry, with burn patients, with children undergoing minor painful procedures, and in obstetrics. Hypnosis can be used to give direct suggestions for pain relief or as an adjunct to psychotherapy or other behavioral treatment.

Unfortunately, not everyone is readily hypnotized, and the best results from using hypnosis to control pain come from patients who are easily hypnotized.

Hypnosis also produces a relaxation response and phenomena unique to hypnosis. These include distorted perceptions, a sense of going back in time, forgetfulness of what happened during the hypnotic episode, and susceptibility to the hypnotist's suggesting a course of action to be followed after hypnosis.

Hypnosis is not just a form of relaxation response. The mechanism underlying hypnosis is not entirely clear. It can be effective in some patients and belongs in the pain-management toolbox.

Biofeedback

We can learn to control our brain-wave activity, to raise or lower our pulse and blood pressure, increase blood supply to one area—such as an arm, with a resultant warming of that hand compared with the other—and relax muscles. Biofeedback helps us modify autonomic nervous system responses. This is the part of the nervous system that automatically controls our minute-to-minute physiology, such as heart rate and blood pressure, without our being aware of it. Biofeedback provides information on these otherwise unconscious biological processes with the goal of giving us control over them. With the help of a trained technician, you are hooked up to electronic instruments that monitor your state of muscle tension, skin temperature, pulse, and brain-wave activity. You can learn to voluntarily control the process, including some that perceive pain.

The basis for biofeedback includes the relaxation response and the work of B. F. Skinner, who showed us that animals can be taught by a system of rewards to control behavior. Biofeedback has been touted as helping many people relax sore muscles and get prolonged benefit in the treatment of recurring tension headaches, migraines, and some muscle pain.

A woman who suffered from back and shoulder pain from tight muscles tried biofeedback. A technician connected electrodes to her neck and shoulders and told her to keep the light green on the attached machine. When the woman's back muscles were relaxed, the light was green. If they tightened, the light became red. The woman could seemingly learn to use her *mind* to keep the green light on so her muscles relaxed. Actually, her *brain* learned to control her body. (Paying attention is important for this learning, but active reasoning is not only unnecessary; it can be counterproductive.)

By paying attention to the lights or other types of feedback from various machines, the woman learns to keep her shoulder and neck muscles relaxed. Once she learns this method, she can continue without the machine, which is the objective. When those who learn to use this method feel a pain coming on, they use what they have learned in biofeed-back to control the muscles that control the pain. Biofeed-back requires trial and error—and a lot of practice.

Psychological Therapy

Another noninterventional treatment on the lower rungs of the pain-management ladder is psychotherapy or behavior therapy. The way you deal psychologically with pain can make you feel like a downtrodden victim, a tough resistance fighter, or somewhere in between. Your approach to dealing with pain may include making a truce with some aspects of it and the limitations it imposes on your functional existence. In the worst case, chronic back pain can make you look at life through glasses tinted with fiery burning red or even black melancholy.

One of the things a good psychotherapist can do is give you strategies to cope with pain, based on who you are, how you were raised, and your earlier experience with pain.

Psychiatrists or psychotherapists skilled at dealing with people in physical pain will focus on practical day-to-day solutions tailored to an individual pain patient. For example, learning to modify or give up an activity to gain pain relief may also allow you to become involved in a satisfying replacement activity.

Since pain may cause depression and anxiety, both of which can in turn increase perceived pain, it may also be useful to take antidepressants and other psychiatric medication as part of the comprehensive treatment (see Chapter 17). Enlisting a psychiatrist who is trained in dealing with patients suffering from chronic pain will also provide access to any necessary psychiatric medication. Physicians who are not psychiatrists should not treat depression or anxiety except in special situations, such as if you lack access to such specialists.

Psychiatrists are medical doctors who know about these medications, their side effects, and their interactions with other drugs. If you do not need psychiatric medication, consider a licensed psychologist or a social worker trained in psychotherapy with experience in dealing with pain.

Key Points about Complementary Therapy for Back Pain

- Various low-risk, low-expense, low–side effect measures may provide pain relief, but in serious pain conditions, such relief may not be of long standing. Repeated treatments are often needed to provide ongoing relief.
- Some types of treatment are not covered by some medical insurers. For example, Medicare does not pay for acupuncture.
- Do not spend months on relaxation training, hypnosis, biofeedback, acupuncture, or spinal manipulation if these methods of treatment do not allow you to graduate to a healthier, less painful state of being, independent of ongoing treatment.
- Alternative and complementary treatments usually cannot hurt you, but that is no reason to undergo treatment that is ineffective in relieving your pain.
- In mild to moderately painful conditions, if after two months these treatments are ineffective, seek another form of therapy.

Part IV

Preventing Back Pain

Chapter 21

Watch Your Back!
How Lifestyle Can Hurt or Help

Common sense and moderation appear at times to be antithetical to the fast pace of the information age. Yet they are the most important ingredients of any program designed to prevent back pain. You are reading this book for one reason: You or someone you know is in pain, and you want to know what can be done about it. Much of the book tells about what may cause pain and how to treat it. Before you have it treated, see if you are causing pain with poor posture or sleep positions, the way you use your body at work or play, or by the amount of weight your spine must support.

The idea of prevention is only just beginning to make a dent in the American psyche. People are giving up smoking despite continued encouragement from the tobacco companies that counteract that attempt by, for instance, sending cases of free cigarettes to the rescue workers at Ground Zero after 9/11. Fast-food chains are now offering salads and lower-fat menu items along with their supersize portions of fat and carbohydrates. Some businesses have installed gyms for their employees or offer incentives such as airline miles to stay fit. Mind you, the bottom line is part of this generosity:

the healthier the employees, the lower the cost of their medical benefits. And one good thing about today's health-care system is that many people who are insured can get screenings to help identify a serious disease early enough to treat it. You can do the same thing to prevent back pain and spinal deterioration by using the proper body mechanics and improving your posture.

In developing nations like India, where some workers carry heavy loads on their backs (or even heads), they sing or chant as they do it. This gives them a rhythm to work in so that they are slow and regular in their movements, not quick or jerky. Sudden lifting or any sudden movement is what gets us into trouble. In this country, a law associate sits twelve hours a day and then runs to get in a two-hour squash game without warming up or mentally and physically relaxing before the game. That's a great prescription for developing back problems. A day laborer in India, despite his physically hard life, may have a healthier back.

You will work longer, harder, and more productively if you take the time to be fit. During the more complicated pain-relieving surgical procedures I perform, I may stand for two to three hours at a time in one place, finish the procedure, and, within twenty minutes, begin another, and finally a third. We are not meant to do this. If you stand a lot, as I do, shift from hip to hip to avoid bursitis and back pain. Don't be a weekend athletic warrior or think you're going to redesign your own garden along the lines of Versailles in one weekend. Athletics and gardens are pleasures of life. Anyone—urbanite, suburbanite, even rural dweller—needs such activities. Moderation is the important word in the lesson. Warm up even before weeding. Someone who exercises in moderation every day is less likely to get hurt than someone who does it only on weekends. Dragging fifty pounds of peat moss on the weekend after spending your week at a desk can precipitate a tear or significant strain in the supporting structures of your back. No matter what you do for a living, your body is your instrument, for yourself and for your family. Take care of it. It can't always be fixed to be as good as new. And you can't turn it in for a new one when the lease runs out or when the repairs have become prohibitively expensive. Here are some commonsense rules.

AVOIDING EXCESS

The athletic prowess that many middle-aged people developed in their youth may now pose a lifestyle dilemma. These people may have the mind set and even the ability to ski a double black diamond slope, even in bad conditions, speeding down at 40 mph or more. However, their bodies may not go along with the ride so forgivingly, especially for the weekend or ski-vacation athlete. Do you ever notice how elegantly and well older ski instructors ski, even down those demanding slopes? Many excellent younger skiers pass them. So what? The trick is to do it enjoyably and well and to be able to keep on doing it, whether your livelihood depends on it or not. Remember: common sense and moderation.

Highly competitive rough sports, pounding sports, or potentially dangerous sports (horseback riding, mountain climbing, gymnastics, skydiving, to name a few) can be psychologically and physically rewarding, but they also can cause lifelong painful injuries. Regular *moderate* exercise is safe, beneficial, and even necessary to a life of vitality and vigor.

I gave up expedition-style mountain climbing for one reason and one reason alone. The summer of the year before I was planning to climb Mount Denali in Alaska, I awoke one morning with a damaged disk in my neck and soon developed pain and weakness in my left arm. I got better without surgery, and the disk shrank to some extent, but it took several months. (I had two closed MRIs—and I am somewhat claustrophobic.) To this day, if I overdo it with that arm, carry heavy loads for a long time, or don't sleep quite right, I feel some pain in my shoulder or arm. It always gets better, but I'm careful. I can't afford to be part of a major climb and have to bail out, letting my fellow climbers or myself down, if that disk horribly declares itself at an inopportune moment, two-thirds of the way up a major peak.

WARM UP FIRST

One of my patients is a garbage collector who gets up early. On winter mornings he makes his rounds seated in a warm truck, but he periodically must step outside into the cold and abruptly lift large, heavy cans with no warm-up. One morning he rose quickly from a bent position to lift a heavy can, injured some of his lumbar facets, and developed an annular tear in a lower lumbar disk, which caused excruciating pain, laying him up for several weeks. (I would like to recommend to the Department of Sanitation that workers start their day by doing warm-up exercises followed by calisthenics.)

Warm up before any physical activity, even regular ones. In warm-ups, the heart rate gradually goes up and muscles get more blood. Muscles, tendons, and ligaments should be stretched before stressing them.

I try to be careful to always warm up, stretch, and cool down before and after athletics. If I haven't exercised in a while because of travel, work, or illness, I start up again slowly. Most joggers know how to stretch before and after exercise. Watch them. They stretch the muscles of the lower back, abdomen, groin, and those that are in the front and back of the legs, using flexion and extension of the muscles in question. The neck, arm, and shoulder muscles can be stretched the same way. Obviously, you should warm up and stretch whatever you are going to use in your exercise routine or sport.

DEVELOP A POSTUREPEDIC BODY

Asked what their motivation was for trying to improve their posture, half the people interviewed by a women's magazine said it was to reduce back pain. Good idea. Posture has a great deal to do with how your back feels. For example, if you keep your head bent forward, you will pull your shoulders forward, too. You will also have neck aches. A potbelly will pull your spine out of alignment and force a slouching posture as well as backache. Stand tall, sit straight, lift with your legs, and never twist and stretch at the same time. Keep your head up and shoulders back. These postures, as you will see below, will help keep your back pain-free.

Being Upright

Standing in one position for a long time tires the muscles in your lower back. You may have experienced this feeling at a cocktail party, in a museum, or at a shopping center. The upright posture increases the curve in the lumbar spine and stretches the muscle in the front of the spine that travels to the hip. Lift one leg and rest it on a stool. Transfer weight from foot to foot or flatten your back with a pelvic tilt (see Chapter 16). These take pressure off the muscles and the curve of your back. Do this any time you stand for a prolonged period, such as when ironing, giving a lecture, or, like me, performing surgical procedures.

When carrying heavy or awkward objects, use both arms. Don't carry things on just one side of your body. In Manhattan, where I work, most people don't have cars. They lug an outrageous amount of things in shoulder bags or backpacks and in the crooks of their arms. Women have taken to staving off dehydration by carrying one or two quarts of water around with them in Manhattan—an excessive amount, especially considering that a quart weighs more than two pounds. And that's not all they carry in their purses, not to mention briefcases. Now I ask you, does that load, usually distributed poorly between the two arms, seem like a good idea if you want to avoid or relieve a spine problem? Similarly, a man carrying a little child behind his head on his neck risks muscular pain and possible cervical-disk herniation.

Lift with Your Legs

When you lift anything, face the object, bend your hips and knees, and lift with your legs, not your back. Keep the object as close to your body as possible. If you must frequently lift heavy objects, consider using an abdominal corset to increase intraabdominal pressure to support your spine. A recent study showed that most people who are given instructions about using abdominal corsets nevertheless use them incorrectly. However, a support may be helpful, even if loosely applied, if it makes you remember to lift with your legs, not your back.

Stretch, Don't Twist

Many of us get into trouble when we stretch. Twisting while stretching is double trouble. On a plane, you have to stretch to squeeze your carry-on bag between heavy suitcases into the overhead bin. Maybe a bag of groceries has shifted to the farthest recesses of your car trunk. In these situations, you may have to stretch to reach, only to recognize that you are about a foot too short for the task! Five seconds later, the muscles in your low back and side have realized this, too, and are now in spasm.

Back pain frequently occurs when you lift even a minimal weight while in a twisted posture. When the spine twists, the muscles are stretched on one side and short on the other. As a result, they are unable to generate the usual support symmetrically around the spine. In this condition, the facets, ligaments, and disks of the back are unnaturally compressed, pushed, and pulled, and the added pressure of lifting a weight only compounds the problem. Inappropriate lifting courts a chronic back problem, which may lead to disk surgery or even a fusion.

The simple answer to overstretching is to get closer to the object you want to move. If it is above your head, get a step stool. (If it's in an airplane's overhead bin, ask for help from a taller person.) Instead of bending over to vacuum, kneel, thus keeping your back straight. Place packages in the front of the trunk or in the back seat.

Sit Straight

Couch potatoes and computer geeks beware. Our lives have evolved to make us more sedentary, but our bodies have not adjusted to the change. Humans were not designed to sit for long periods. Get up and move periodically. When you sit, use a chair that offers back support. The gothic church chair is better for your back than all of these high-tech ergonomic extravaganzas that are claimed to be comfortable.

The best chair for anyone with back pain is one with a firm upholstered seat, a firm straight back, and armrests. In a soft chair, your back is constantly making adjustments to support your spine. These tiny adjustments can cause fatigue or increase pain because your back is working very hard.

When you sit in a chair with firm support, the muscles can relax because the chair supports them.

The seat depth should support your entire thigh, and the height should allow you to place your feet flat on the floor with your knees slightly higher than your hips. Chairs used in offices have an adjustable back and wheels. The tension and position of the back support should be adjustable as should the height of the seat. If you need more lumbar support, roll up a bath towel and put it behind the small of your back.

Try a kneeler chair to see if it relieves back pain.

Stand Up Periodically

If you have a desk job, you can easily fall into the trap of being so engrossed in your computer screen that hours go by, and you move nothing but your fingers on the keyboard and your eyes on the screen.

Get up once in a while. If you can't remember, set a timer for thirty minutes to tell you to get up and stretch. Roll your head around to stretch your neck. Lift your arms into the air and stretch. Put your hands on your hips and bend your body forward, backward, and from side to side. Jump up and down in place. Whatever you do, you periodically need to change from the seated position to give your spine a break. (See the advice in the travel section below about what to do if you are seated in a car for long periods.)

Sleep Soundly

People often ask me what kind of mattress they should have. Quite honestly, I don't know or care; whatever works. Get a mattress that you—and your significant other, if there is one—like. Does a good mattress improve your spine? I'm not sure it can alter your anatomy, but it can certainly give you a better night's sleep. The more you toss and turn, the worse it is for your neck.

Cricks in the neck. The neck is most often injured during sleep when you toss and turn, thus increasing pressure on the disks of the neck. Many cervical-disk herniations are sensed when you awaken, not when you try to lift something. An early description of the cervical disk was made by a Memphis neurosurgeon. He had a patient, a farmer, who awoke one morning with a crick in his neck that continued down his arm. The pain was persistent and bad enough that he sought medical help and ended up seeing the neurosurgeon. The details of the rest of the story aren't important here. The onset of a cervical-disk herniation is. I'm not sure how effectively a cervical-disk herniation can be prevented by proper nighttime positioning, but a few ideas come to mind. I do believe your nighttime position influences your pain and recovery—or lack thereof—from a cervical-disk herniation.

If you have neck problems, make an effort to sleep on your back, even if it is hard to do. Pillows are important. Use a good pillow, one that is soft enough to keep your neck from severely arching and large and hard enough to raise your head slightly to shoulder level. I am not convinced that cervical pillows are a good means of relieving neck pain for all people. If you have one and feel it helps you, by all means use it. However, many of these therapeutic pillows, like traveling pillows, make you arch your neck and put more pressure on the disks and facets in the neck.

Low-back pain. Don't sleep on your stomach. It twists your neck and increases the backward curve of your lumbar spine, potentially causing more pain. If you have to sleep on your stomach, put a pillow or two under your abdomen.

This will flatten your spine and place less pressure on the pelvic muscles.

Get in and out of bed carefully if you have back pain. Push yourself up with your lower arm while sliding your legs off the edge of the bed. The weight of your legs will swing your chest up with the support of your arm against the bed. Do the reverse to get back into bed. Shift your upper body weight to the palm of the hand that's resting on the bed. Slowly lower your body, shifting your weight to your forearm, elbow, and shoulder while you swing your legs up onto the bed. Try to keep your back straight.

WATCH YOUR WEIGHT

Most Americans are overweight, a problem that is spreading to Europe, where they have adopted our calorie-laden fast foods and gargantuan portions. The increase in obesity has happened gradually over the past few decades because we not only eat more but we move less. We used to eat three meals a day and do more physical work. Now we eat all the time, not only at home but in the shopping mall, at the movies, and at the ball game. Our work has become less physical. We spend the day in front of a computer then go home and flop on the couch. The overweight problem is most obvious in small towns and suburban areas where people drive everywhere, even to their garbage cans. In cities people walk more, thus fewer are overweight or obese.

Being overweight becomes a chronic disease from which it is increasingly difficult to recover. It also contributes to an enormous number of medical problems, including arthritis, heart disease, diabetes, and cancer.

Excess weight prematurely wears out your musculoskeletal system, causing an accelerated risk of disk herniation and spinal slippage. Both of these conditions lead to surgery—

potentially repeated surgery—in overweight people, in whom these problems are more likely to recur. So by eating poorly and being sedentary, you marry to the medical system. It's a bad marriage, especially for you.

I try to keep within a five-pound range of the appropriate weight for a man of my height. That is not always easy as I get older and am more sedentary than when I was younger. I never snack. I eat a high-quality Mediterranean diet, occasionally including meat and sweets, and drink alcohol (mostly red wine) in moderation. I never eat less than two hours before bedtime. I smoke an occasional cigar or pipe. This regime works well for me. It works well for most of the people in Europe, where I was raised. I am not holding myself up, by any means, as a model to emulate. I do represent a typical person who may have pain (and therefore wants to read this book).

For most people, the body mass index (BMI) is a good measure of whether you are overweight. Guidelines from the National Institutes of Health define overweight as a BMI greater than 25. Obesity starts at a BMI of 30. If you are six feet tall and weigh 200 pounds, your BMI would be 27, which is a bit high. You would be better off weighing 170 to 180.

PREVENT RECURRING BACK PAIN

Strong back muscles represent another type of fitness. Compared with other muscles in the body, the muscles in the back are generally weak. If we can increase strength in these muscles we can reduce our risk of developing back pain. This is important for everyone, and it is critical for those whose jobs require heavy lifting and heavy labor. Exercises that strengthen the muscles in the front (abdominal flexors) and in the back (back extensors) can reduce your risk of injury if you lift heavy objects or twist and bend frequently at work.

Do your general fitness exercises every other day. The day off allows your body to revitalize muscles fatigued by the exercise. Engage in an exercise program vigorous enough to stimulate about twenty to thirty minutes of perspiration. Exercise of this type also improves circulation, bone density, flexibility, and muscle tone.

Don't Smoke

Your lungs are not the only part of your body that is damaged by smoking. All the tissues of the body need oxygen to maintain their function. Smoking keeps them from getting the optimal amount of oxygen. Lack of oxygen is part of the disk-disintegration process that increases the risk of herniation. There are no blood vessels supplying the interior of the disks, so oxygen has to seep in from the surface. If the blood contains less oxygen, the disks receive less, too. Smoking also reduces the likelihood that a fusion will properly heal.

ENJOY PAINFREE TRAVELING

We all travel more than ever before. It can be fun, work, or hell, depending on how you do it and how much pain you are in or develop as a result of doing it. I do think that some precautions may limit travel-related pain.

On Airplanes

- If you have a bad back and fly coach, try to reserve the first seat at the bulkhead, where you have more legroom. For many low-back pain sufferers, sitting up straight usually is preferable.
- If you travel frequently, get a credit card or join a frequent-flyer program that gives you access to an airport lounge, where you can relax in a good chair.

- Don't store heavy objects in overhead racks. Put them on the floor under your seat to avoid the strain of reaching up to pull down an awkward weight.
- When reserving seats in coach, ask for flights that are not completely booked so that you can stretch out in the empty seats. Book your flight well in advance and get the best seat.
- If you have neck problems and are taking a long flight, decide for yourself if a cervical traveling pillow is good for you. It's a function of what's comfortable, not what your doctor says.
- If you take a two-week trip somewhere, consider whether traveling in coach—where you'll be squashed for hours—is really worth the savings, considerable though they may be. It may pay to book a roomier seat that will protect your back so you can enjoy your two-week vacation and be able to return to work afterward so that you can pay for it.
- If you get off the plane and your back hurts, rest, no matter what! If you have a bad back, consider a beach vacation that offers warmth and water.
- Don't drink alcohol or coffee on the flight. These will impair your sleep and exacerbate jet lag, which in turn can further impair your sleep, increase muscle tension, make your pain worse, and interfere with normal daytime activity.
- On planes, trains, and buses, sit on an aisle, where you can move more easily.

Driving
- If you rent a car, check the model to make sure it is comfortable for you and easy to load and unload, in case you are in a pickle in a small

Tuscan town and nobody is around to unload your baggage. Some small cars can be bad for your back.

- The tension of driving and not knowing where you are going is stressful. Nervous tension makes pain worse, and the body becomes more disposed to break down. Know where you're going and how to get there.
- When sitting in a car for extended periods, roll from side to side in your seat. Roll from one side of your backside to the other. Do this every twenty minutes to keep your spine supple. This will reduce or prevent stiffness later, when the trip is over.
- When you get out of the car, roll your neck and shoulders. Place your hands on the back of your head so that your elbows are even with your ears. Then pull your elbows backward as far as they can go. Another one is to clasp your hands behind your buttocks, then roll your shoulders back as you extend your arms out behind you.
- When you drive for long periods, stop every hour or so and walk around. Swing your arms wide and get your blood circulating again. Getting blood into your muscles helps prevent stiffness.
- If your car has an adjustable built-in lumbar support, use it. It may take some experimenting and adjusting to get it just right, but it will certainly make you more comfortable. Of course, it may make you very *un*comfortable if you don't adjust it properly. The same is true for a portable lumbar support you can place on the seat.

Walking and Carrying

- Wear comfortable shoes, ones suitable for what you are doing. If you are walking on unpaved paths in the countryside or for hours on cobblestone streets, you may want an excellent walking shoe or even a light hiking shoe. (Heavy hiking shoes would be overkill.)

- Think ahead to be up to physical demands. If you know that walking causes pain in your low back and you want to visit a museum, take pain medication forty-five minutes before you anticipate needing it so it is already in your body before the pain begins. It works better that way. Don't just pop a pill in your mouth when pain hits; it won't work very well if you do.

- Distribute the weight of what you carry rather than tote everything in one hand. (See how many people in airports carry two suitcases in one hand and a two-ounce ticket in the other.)

- Use rolling luggage with an extendable handle, and attach all your shoulder bags to it.

- Use a carrying cart available in airports or, better yet, find a porter for help. Porters are well worth the expense. They save your spine and can often help expedite you through the ticketing area.

- Tip the cabdriver or van driver explicitly to help you with your luggage. Do not try to be macho. (This goes for women, too.)

- If you carry heavy equipment, such as a camera, balance it on your body as you did with your valises. Special vests for photographers may be helpful.

- Fanny belts—not fashionable urban backpacks, the majority of which are poorly designed for carrying heavy weight—are the best solution for carrying weight for a long period of time.

Sleeping Away from Home

- Spend money on accommodations with a decent bed that will protect your back and enable you to enjoy your vacation.
- Changing time zones can affect your sleep. Organize the first day or two of activities to ease into the new time zone. You may have to stay up later on the day of arrival to get into the sleep pattern of the place to which you have traveled.

Adjusting Medications

- Take extra care to follow the dosing schedules of your medication. Most medications last only three to six hours. If you need lots of pain medicine, reconsider what you're doing and adjust gradually to the pace of wherever you are, allowing for changing time zones. Consider using longer-acting medicine if possible. Test it out well in advance of traveling.
- Depending on your medical history and where you are going, you may want to take medicine to prevent coughing, constipation, and vomiting. These problems can cause disk-related pain or make it worse.

GLOSSARY

Acupuncture: a traditional Chinese therapeutic process in which specific points of the body are stimulated with needles to foster healing or pain relief.

Analgesia: relief of pain.

Anesthesia: loss of sensation; also a treatment that causes controlled analgesia, amnesia (lack of recollection of events) and muscular relaxation.

Annulus: the leathery covering of a disk that surrounds the nucleus, or rubbery core.

Arachnoid: the spiderweb-like covering of the brain, spinal cord, cauda equina, and nerve roots in the spinal canal and inner foramen.

Autonomic nervous system: the part of the nervous system that functions without our conscious awareness regulating heart rate, blood pressure, sweating, and certain aspects of digestion, for example.

Block: an injection of a chemical that blocks the transmission of nerve impulses; used for diagnostic and therapeutic purposes.

Bursa: a fluid-filled sac overlying a joint that reduces friction from the muscles that slide over the joint.

Cauda equina: Latin for horse's tail. A group of nerve roots exiting the end of the spinal cord in the upper lumbar spine. These roots control the muscle power and sensation of the lower extremities and also bowel, bladder, and sexual functions.

Cervical: pertaining to the neck.

Compression fracture: collapse of a vertebral body, caused by trauma or by weakening from osteoporosis or cancer.

Congenital: a condition existing from birth.

Corticosteroids: man-made analogues of hormones produced by the adrenal glands that affect various bodily systems. They possess potent anti-inflammatory and pain-relieving properties and have considerable side effects.

CT scan: a diagnostic radiological technique using a computer to deliver three-dimensional pictures of internal organs, including the spine.

Decompression surgery: spinal surgery to relieve the pressure of a neurological structure: spinal cord or nerve root.

Discectomy: a surgical procedure to remove disk material that has become displaced outside the annulus by a disk herniation.

Discogenic: originating in a disk, as in discogenic pain.

Discogram: a procedure to determine which disks are causing pain. Radiological dye is injected into a disk, and the patient's response is observed. If the injection reproduces a patient's pain, the disk is considered a source of discogenic pain. A discogram also reveals the structural condition of the interior of the disk and its covering.

Disk: flattened circular structure, something like a checker piece, with a firm rubbery core and leathery covering called the annulus. Disks lie between the vertebral bodies of the spine.

Dorsal: pertaining to the back of the body; a dorsal root enters the back of the spinal cord.

Dura: the tough external covering of the brain, spinal cord, cauda equina, and nerve roots. Under the dura are the arachnoid, spinal fluid, and nervous system structures.

Electromyogram (EMG): an electrical diagnostic test, usually combined with a nerve conduction velocity (NCV) examination. Together they are used to evaluate disorders of the spinal nerve roots, peripheral nerves, and muscles.

Epidural: pertaining to the area within the spinal canal outside the dura. It contains fat and veins.

Facet: a joint stabilizing the spine. Facets are located on either side of the spine and connect a vertebra to the one above and the one below.

Facetectomy: spinal surgery to remove part of a facet.

Fascia: a layer of connective tissue that surrounds the muscles.

Fibromyalgia: a painful condition characterized by tender areas within the muscles in widespread areas. It is not to be confused with myofascial pain, which occurs in smaller focal areas of muscle tenderness.

Fluoroscopy: an X-ray device that provides live images to a physician during placement of needles and electrodes to areas of the body.

Foramen (plural: foramina): holes on either side of the vertebrae through which the spinal roots exit the spinal canal.

Foramenotomy: spinal surgery that widens the foramen to relieve pressure on a nerve root passing through it.

Fusion: spinal surgery to fuse together one or more vertebrae.

Ganglion (plural: ganglia): a mass of cell bodies of sensory or autonomic nerves. Each spinal root and some cranial nerves (leaving the brain) have a ganglion. There are various autonomic ganglia near the spine and in other parts of the body.

Herniate: the projection of tissue (disk, muscle, intestine) through a defect in surrounding tissue. In disk herniation, the rubbery core of the disk pushes through the annulus. Sometimes, not always, this material presses on a nerve and causes pain.

Horse's tail: See cauda equina.

Intraspinal: inside the spinal canal. In this book, it refers to drug delivery into either the epidural space or spinal fluid.

Intrathecal: inside the covering containing the spinal fluid.

Lamina: one of the two sides of the arch arising from the back of the vertebral body. The arch makes up the back of the spinal canal.

Laminectomy: removal of both arches of a vertebra.

Laminotomy: removal of part of one arch of a vertebra.

Lesioning: partial or complete destruction of nerve tissue. In this book, lesions are made for the purpose of stopping or moderating the pain messages sent by those nerves to the brain.

Ligamentum flavum: Latin for yellow ligament. These are the ligaments inside the spinal canal that stabilize the spine. With age, they bulge and become hard with calcium deposits, thus causing narrowing of the spinal canal and exerting pressure on the nerve roots.

Lumbar: having to do with the lower spine between the lowest rib and the pelvis.

MRI (magnetic resonance imaging): a diagnostic technique that provides two-dimensional images of the structure of the body by exposure to a magnetic field. It does not use radiation.

Musculoskeletal: pertaining to ligaments, tendons, muscle, and bone. Musculoskeletal pain occurs in these structures and accompanies most back pain and many disorders.

Myelogram: a diagnostic test in which radiological dye is injected into the spinal fluid; X-rays and later CT scans are taken to evaluate sources of pressure on the spinal cord and nerve roots (such as disk herniations, stenosis, and spinal slippage).

Myofascial pain: pain in areas of muscle contraction.

Narcotics: a class of drug that binds to specific receptors in the body that are also bound to by endorphins, its naturally occurring narcotic-like chemicals. Narcotics may be used to relieve moderate-to-severe pain.

Neuralgia: pain traveling along the course of a nerve or nerves that is caused by dysfunction or damage to the nerve or nerves.

Neurogenic claudication: pain in the legs caused by pressure from stenosis within the spine on the nerve roots that control nerves to the legs. Claudication is induced by exercise and relieved by rest, either sitting or lying down.

Neuropathic: pertaining to pain or unpleasant sensation caused by nervous-system dysfunction or injury.

NSAIDs (nonsteroidal anti-inflammatory drugs): a type of painkilling drug that reduces inflammation. They block the production of prostaglandins, chemicals that cause inflammation and initiate pain. Aspirin is the most common NSAID.

Nucleus: the rubbery central portion of a disk.

Pain: an unpleasant sensory or emotional experience, not necessarily a result of damage to the body.

Radicular pain: caused by root irritation or dysfunction.

Radiofrequency: a type of energy that can be harnessed to produce heat. With appropriate equipment, it can be used to achieve partial or complete destruction of tissue, including nerve tissue.

Referred pain: pain transmitted to an area distant from its cause.

Root: the portion of a nerve running between the spinal cord and foramen. Once the root exits the foramen, it is simply called a nerve. Roots are also referred to as spinal roots or nerve roots.

Sciatica: a nonmedical layman's term referring to pain from the low back or buttock that travels down the leg. It is a symptom, not a condition.

Spinal canal: the space within the spine through which course the spinal cord, roots, and their coverings. It is composed of the arches of the vertebrae.

Spinal cord: the part of the central nervous system extending from the base of the brain down to the upper lumbar spine. It serves to bring messages (sensations) about the body from the roots up to the brain and bring messages from the brain down to the roots, from which they travel to the peripheral nerves.

Spinal fluid: a clear, colorless, waterlike fluid that bathes the spinal cord and brain.

Spine: the column of bones, disks, and ligaments running from the base of the skull to the pelvis that encloses the spinal cord, cauda equina, and nerve roots.

Spinous process: the mildly bony protuberance, or row of bumps, in the back of the vertebrae felt or seen under the skin in thin people.

Spondylitis: inflammation of the joints (facets and disks) connecting the vertebrae.

Spondyloarthropathy: a disease of the joints of the spine.

Spondylolisthesis: occurs when one vertebral body slips over another.

Spondylolysis: a defect in the formation of the L_5 vertebra that can lead to spinal instability.

Spondylosis: also known as stenosis; an acquired arthritic narrowing of the spinal canal.

Stenosis: narrowing of the spinal canal or foramina from arthritic overgrowth, disk bulges or herniation, bulging ligaments, or spinal slippage. In some people, the canal is already narrow at birth (congenital stenosis).

Tender points: See myofascial pain.

TENS (transcutaneous electrical nerve stimulation): a pain-relieving therapy in which mild electrical stimulation from a portable device is delivered to the skin through small electrodes glued to it.

Test-negative pain: pain that has no cause that can be detected by plain X-rays, CT scans, MRI, electrical tests, or laboratory-based diagnostic tools. It may be investigated with diagnostic nerve blocks and discograms.

Thoracic: pertaining to the chest area, or that part of the spine to which the ribs are attached.

Trigger point: a small knotted bundle of fibers within a muscle that is the cause of myofascial muscle pain.

Vertebra (plural: vertebrae): a bone of the spine in part composed of the vertebral body, lamina, and facets.

Vertebral bodies: the supporting part of a vertebra in the front of the spine that takes the greatest weight. Disks are located between the vertebral bodies.

Vertebroplasty: a procedure in which liquefied orthopedic bone cement is injected into partially collapsed pain-generating bones (usually vertebral bodies) with the intent of relieving the otherwise poorly controlled pain. It is especially beneficial to patients suffering from painful vertebral fractures caused by osteoporosis or cancer.

Yellow ligament: See ligamentum flavum.

APPENDIX

Information Resources

American Academy of Orthopedic Surgeons
6300 North River Road
Rosemont IL 60018
phone: 800 346-2267
website: www.aaos.org

American Academy of Pain Management
13947 Mono Way #A
Sonora CA 95370
phone: 209 533-9744
email: aapm@aapainmanage.org
website: www.aapainmanage.org

American Chronic Pain Association
POB 850
Rocklin CA 95677
phone: 800 533-3231
website: www.theacpa.org

American Massage Therapy Association
820 Davis Street
Evanston IL 60201
phone: 847 864-0123
website: www.amtamassage.org

American Pain Foundation
211 North Charles Street, Suite 710
Baltimore MD 21201
website: www.painfoundation.org

American Physical Therapy Association
1111 North Fairfax Street
Alexandria VA 22314
phone: 800 999-2782
website: www.apta.org

Arthritis Foundation
1330 West Peachtree Street
Atlanta GA 30309
phone: 800 283-7800
email: help@arthritis.org
website: www.arthritis.org

Back Pain Association of America
POB 135
Pasadena MD 21122-0135
phone: 410 255-3633
email: backpainassoc@fmsn.com

Cancer Care
275 Seventh Avenue
New York NY 10001
phone: 212 221-3300 or 800 813-4673
email: info@cancercare.org
website: www.cancercare.org

International Association for the Study of Pain
909 NE Forty-third Street, Suite 306
Seattle WA 98105-6020
website: www.iasp-pain.org

National Foundation for the Treatment of Pain
POB 70045
Houston TX 77270
phone: 713 862-9332
website: www.paincare.org

National Institutes of Health
Bethesda MD 20892
phone: 301 496-4000
website: www.nih.gov

Spondylitis Association of America
POB 5872
Sherman Oaks CA 91413
phone: 800 777-8189
website: www.spondylitis.org

INDEX

Page numbers in *italics* refer to illustrations.